"Drs. Wen and Kosowsky have insightfully crafted a revelation about the workings of modern medicine. It addresses with a finely nuanced balance the basis for our dysfunctional 'cookbook style' of medicine. The analysis is not a critical pontification by outsiders, but a pained view by deeply informed insiders. The book pleads powerfully for the disenfranchised patient. It must be read both because most of us sooner or later are bound to seek health care and because the authors provide an important viewpoint for the intensifying nationwide health care debate."

—Bernard Lown, M.D., Professor Emeritus, Harvard School
of Public Health; Senior Physician Emeritus Brigham &
Women's Hospital; Nobel Peace Laureate 1985

"A powerful appeal for individualized medical evaluation based on an active partnership between doctors and patients. The rational, mutual approach to diagnosis advocated by Drs. Wen and Kosowsky is the antidote for mindless and wasteful routines that all too often replace careful listening and focused assessment of each patient."

—Harvey V. Fineberg, M.D., Ph.D., president, Institute of Medicine

"Wen and Kosowsky have revisited the never-ending debate around the 'art and science of medicine' hoping to strike the right balance in the practice of emergency health care. Their hands-on discussion of the limits of algorithmic medicine is precise and timely. Their proposal for "diagnostic partnership" is a major contribution of this courageous book in which common sense plays the leading role."

—Julio Frenk, M.D., Ph.D., dean of the
Harvard School of Public Health

"Drs. Wen and Kosowsky propose an innovative approach to fixing U.S. healthcare that begins with the patient. Read this book and now you—as a patient—can be the change our country has been waiting for."

—Elliot S. Fisher, M.D., M.P.H., director of
Population Health and Policy, The Dartmouth Institute

"Using real patient examples, Drs. Wen and Kosowsky paint a disturbing portrait of medicine gone awry and provide a simple series of prescriptions to empower patients to get their health care back on track."

—Ron M. Walls, M.D., professor and chair, Department of Emergency
Medicine, Brigham & Women's Hospital, Harvard Medical School

"A wake-up call to move beyond cookbook American medicine to a new medical practice that brings the humanity back into the core of the 'art' of healing."
—Lincoln C. Chen, M.D., director, Global Equity Center at Harvard Kennedy School of Government

"In this era of overweening medical technology, doctors and their patients are a great risk of losing touch with the centrality of 'patient-centered' care. *When Doctors Don't Listen* not only offers a compelling argument for revitalizing this touchstone of good medicine, but also provides a comprehensive guide for how doctors and patients can improve the quality of healthcare by doing so."
—Jordan J. Cohen, M.D., professor of medicine and public health, George Washington University; president emeritus, Association of American Medical Colleges

"This is an important contribution to helping both physicians and patients more effectively manage their encounters."
—Robert Graham, M.D., professor of family and community medicine, University of Cincinnati

"This book is a must-read for informing the dialogue about healthcare reform and transforming medical education. . . . The authors' passion for the individual behind the illness is contagious. . . . Their argument for bringing back the value of clinical judgment is brilliantly written, and is amply supported with case studies. In many ways this is a book about the humanism of the physician as much as it is about patients as human beings."
—Afaf I. Meleis, Ph.D., DrPS (hon), FAAN, Margaret Bond Simon Dean of Nursing, University of Pennsylvania School of Nursing

"Drs. Leana Wen and Joshua Kosowsky make the case that the resultant algorithms-gone-wild syndrome seen in many medical settings today actually drives imprecise and wasteful testing, muddled diagnoses, and patient confusion. They argue that these clinical behaviors are at the heart of our 'morbidly obese' medical care system and that thoughtful physicians relying on patient narratives and diagnostic common sense will create a leaner medical care system and better patient outcomes. Theirs is a contrarian and compelling case with the well-being of millions of patients and $250 billion a year riding on it."
—Fitzhugh Mullan, M.D., Murdock Head Professor of Medicine and Health Policy, George Washington University

"What a brilliant concept—this outstanding book provides an innovative and interesting approach to understanding how physicians interact with patients . . . This excellent book contains a literal treasure trove of information which will be beneficial and educational for patient and physician alike."

—W. Brian Gibler, M.D. FACEP, FACC, president and CEO, University Hospital; senior vice president, UC Health; professor of emergency medicine, University of Cincinnati College of Medicine

"A commonsense and deeply sincere prescription to help patients advocate for their own health."

—Sandeep Jauhar, M.D., author of *Intern: A Doctor's Initiation.*

"Doctors take an oath to do no harm. Yet more than ever, modern medicine makes healthy people sick. Emergency physicians Leana Wen and Josh Kosowsky make a passionate argument for patients to get involved and informed about their care. A fast, smart read to help you take charge of your health."

—Audrey Young Crissman, M.D., author of *What My Patients Taught Me. A Medical Student's Journey*

When Doctors Don't Listen

How to Avoid Misdiagnoses and Unnecessary Tests

Leana Wen, M.D.

and Joshua Kosowsky, M.D.

Thomas Dunne Books
St. Martin's Press ⚏ New York

This book is dedicated to
Leana's mother,
Sandy Ying Zhang (1954–2010),
whose long struggle with cancer was an inspiration for the book,
and to all of our patients, for teaching us, guiding us, and allowing
us to practice the art and science of medicine.

THOMAS DUNNE BOOKS.
An imprint of St. Martin's Press.

www.thomasdunnebooks.com
www.stmartins.com

ISBN 978-0-312-59491-6 (hardcover)
ISBN 978-1-250-01357-6 (e-book)

First Edition: January 2013

10 9 8 7 6 5 4 3 2 1

Acknolwedgments

There are many people who were instrumental in turning this book from idea into reality. We would like to thank our agent, Jessica Papin, for believing in us from the start. Jessica, your confidence in us never waivered, and we could not have done this project without your sage advice and your expert guidance. Similarly, we are indebted to our editor, Rob Kirkpatrick, his assistant Nicole Sohl, our publicist Joan Higgins, and the rest of the excellent team at Thomas Dunne Books/St. Martin's Press. Their influence can be seen, literally, on every page.

As this is a book about the practice of medicine, we must also thank those clinical and research mentors who have guided us throughout the years. These remarkable individuals include: Dr. James Adams, Dr. John Atkinson, Dr. David Brown, Dr. Carlos Camargo, Dr. Hal Churchill, Dr. Raymond Garcia, Dr. Brian Gibler, Dr. Leslie Kahl, Dr. Bernard Lown, Dr. Fitzhugh Mullan, Dr. Donald Paulson, Dr. William Peck, Dr. Ron Wallo, and Paul R. Wright.

We also thank the many expert clinicians, health-policy experts, and health writers who have helped us with this book: Dr. Stephen Bergman, Dr. Howard Blumstein, Ms. Shannon Brownlee, Dr. Doug Char, Dr. Lincoln Chen, Dr. Jordan Cohen, Dr. Audrey Young Crissman, Dr. James Ducharme, Dr. Harvey Fineberg, Dr. Elliot Fischer, Dr. Julio Frenk, Dr. Sandeep Jauhar,

Dr. Robert Graham, Dr. Jerome Hoffman, Dr. Robert McNamara, Dr. Afaf Meleis, Dr. Siddhartha Mukerjee, Dr. Fitzhugh Mullan, Dr. Jesse Pines, Dr. Ali Raja, Dr. Mark Reiter, Dr. Lisa Sanders, Dr. Darshak Sanghavi, Dr. Ian Stiell, Dr. Ben Sun, Dr. Ron Walls, Dr. Mark Weinstock, and Dr. Larry Weiss.

Breast cancer survivors and outspoken activists Melissa Etheridge and Fran Drescher have been central to our book promotion, and we thank them for their continuing efforts to advocate for patients and for joining us in our movement to empower patients.

A number of individuals provided comments and edits to improve early drafts of the book. We acknowledge the time and efforts of Dr. Seth Bloom, Noam Broder, Michael Cannon, Genevieve Quist Green, Dr. Edith Gurrola, Brian Johnsrud, Shirley Mertz, Amber Price, Katrina Roi, and Vivian Sisskin.

We want to thank our colleagues. Leana has learned so much from her medical school and residency classmates and attendings and from the nurses, physician assistants, and other staff at Brigham & Women's Hospital and Massachusetts General. Josh is grateful to his colleagues at Brigham & Women's Hospital and his students at Harvard Medical School.

Many thanks to our close friends who supported us through the process of conceiving and writing our book. Leana wishes to thank Erin Brooks, Lyric Chen, Dr. Kao-Ping Chua, Sara Deon, Christo Fogelberg, Dr. Yvonne Fulbright, Brian Johnsrud, Jeff Marlow, Chase Mendenhall, Aaron Mertz, Dr. Griffin Myers, Dr. Jonathan Rogg, Dr. Neel Shah, Ryan Thoreson, Grace Vesom, Dr. Jonathan Welch, and Pia Wojtinnek. They have heard her go on and on for three years about this book, and they deserve credit for their patience and never-ending support. Josh thanks Gary Belsky, Dr. Hal Blumenfeld, Dr. Stephen Bohan, Dr. Jay Harris, Brian Yablon, and Dr. Richard Zane.

Then there are our families, who endured many late nights and endless discussions with us. We are grateful to our spouses, Sebastian Walker and Devorah Kosowsky. Thanks to Leana's sister, Angela Wen, father, Xiaolu Wen, and most of all, to her mother, Sandy, who passed away while this book was being written. It was from her that Leana learned the most important lessons of compassion and humanism. Josh's parents, Joyce and Dr.

Bernard Kosowsky, have been steadfast in their encouragement and support throughout his career. Some of Josh's earliest memories are of stories of patients and doctors (including Dr. Lown!) told around the dinner table. To this day, Josh looks up to his father as the clinician *par excellence*. He is also grateful to his children, Harry, Jake, and Judah, who are a continual source of joy and inspiration.

Last, but certainly not least, we thank our patients. It is for you, our patients and our readers that we write this book. We thank you for your patience and acceptance of us as doctors, the new doctors-in-training as well as the "older" doctors who are continuing to refine our practice. We continue to learn so much from you every day. We are excited to join together on this journey to improve medical care and to reaffirm what medicine is about: to serve patients and to serve society.

Authors' Note

The stories contained within this are based on our true experiences as doctors in the Emergency Room (ER). In order to protect patient confidentiality, patient names and characteristics have been changed throughout the book. In some incidences, composite characters have been used and the time sequence has been altered. Any resemblance to real-life individuals is purely coincidental. Physician names, when disclosed, are accurate.

Contents

Introduction

One Friday afternoon, Jerry Robertson got the scare of his life.

Jerry is a forty-eight-year-old mechanic who knows each of his customers as well as he knows their cars. "To understand the car, you gotta understand the driver," he likes to say. He sports a well-worn Red Sox cap, but his vowels betray his "New Yawk" roots.

To see his 250-pound frame and round belly now, you wouldn't guess that Jerry spent hours at the pool every day in high school and was something of a star swimmer. The time he devoted to athletics now goes to running his garage, providing for his wife and three children, and, once in a blue moon, "drinking beer and playing pokers with the guys." His health was never really an issue. "I know I'm a little out of shape and I gotta lose some weight," he admits, but otherwise he's always felt just fine.

All of that changed unexpectedly one weekend last July. His younger brother, the eternal bachelor, had finally decided to move in with his girlfriend. Friday was the big day, and Jerry was recruited to help with this momentous occasion. "For a single guy, you sure have accumulated a lot of crap," Jerry had remarked. "And heavy crap, too!" After eight solid hours of lifting, squatting, carrying, and lugging—interrupted only by the twenty-minute U-Haul drive across town—the two brothers called it quits and celebrated with a trip to the local pub.

Saturday morning, Jerry woke up with tightness in his chest. It hurt when he sat up and he figured he must have pulled something while he was moving. But his uncle or grandfather (maybe both?) had heart problems, and Jerry's wife persuaded him to go to the ER to get it checked out.

A generation ago, a doctor might have heard Jerry's story and told him that he had a muscle strain. He would have left and felt better. Not so on this particular day. The nurse who greeted Jerry noted his "chief complaint" of chest pain and called over a tech, who took off Jerry's shirt and attached him to a monitor that beeped and displayed waves and numbers that made no sense to him, but Jerry trusted the folks around him to make sense of it all. He was given some aspirin to chew and another tiny pill under his tongue that tingled a bit and gave him a headache. He was brought to a treatment room where another nurse came in and asked a series of questions about his "chest pain" before proceeding to take several vials of blood and shuttling him off to the next destination, the radiology suite for X-rays. When he finally got back, a doctor stopped in and went over yet another checklist of questions, these seeming even less relevant to why he was there. ("Why did it matter whether I had blood in my stool or slept on two pillows at night?") But while long, convoluted, and confusing for Jerry, the whole process nevertheless appeared routine and procedural for the ensemble of medical professionals coming and going.

Hours passed. Finally, the doctor in charge (we'll call him Dr. M.) came in and told Jerry that everything looked fine so far, but that he needed to stay overnight for some more tests.

Jerry didn't want to stay. He had already missed his son's hockey game; he didn't want to miss his daughter's choir performance, too.

"Why can't I go home? I'm not having a heart attack, am I?" he asked.

"Probably not, but we can't be sure," Dr. M. replied. "That's what the 'chest pain pathway' is for."

Jerry felt trapped. If there was a chance he could be having a heart attack, he couldn't exactly go, could he? If the heart pains didn't kill him, his wife *definitely* would if she found out he'd skipped off the trail of this so-called "chest pain pathway" that the doctor was leading him down. So he dutifully stayed the night. The next morning, he was relieved when they told him that he hadn't, in fact, had a heart attack. That was good news, but his ordeal wasn't over. Dr. M. told him that they still could not be sure what was caus-ing his chest pain or confirm there weren't problems with his heart. The test that monitored him running on a treadmill was "nondiagnostic"—he couldn't run as much as they needed him to, so the test couldn't show a re-sult, one way or the other.

"You should see your primary care doctor to follow up on this," Dr. M. cautioned. "He'll probably want to order some more advanced tests."

Jerry went home, far from reassured and more confused than ever. Why did Dr. M. make it sound like he had something bad? If he didn't have a heart attack, what could it be? Was it cancer? His father had died of lung cancer in his early fifties, but he was a heavy smoker. Why couldn't someone have told him what was really going on? His chest was still a little sore and it got worse after the kids pounced on him when he got home . . . should he be worried about this? Can he keep working, what with crawling under all those cars? Is he going to be OK?

Healthcare reform dominates today's discussions. Every day, our airwaves are inundated with the latest political debates on how to increase healthcare access while reducing costs. What is rarely discussed is how patients are increasingly dissatisfied by their lack of meaningful participation in their own medical care. What is not mentioned is how medicine has morphed from thoughtful engagement between doctors and patients to cookie-cutter recipes that regard all individuals alike. And how this **cookbook approach,** defined by its rote and formulaic approach to practicing medicine, leads to less accurate diagnoses—and worse outcomes—for patients. But is Dr. M to blame for relying on a way of thinking, that has been taught and reinforced among doctors for a generation or more?

It used to be that people went to their doctor to find out what was wrong. That was the expectation when someone made an appointment with their local family doctor: they wanted to know what they had and how they could feel better. Ear infection: what should I take? Pulled muscle: what should I do? Broken ankle: how can you fix it?

Over the years, something happened to this common sense approach. "Algorithms" and "pathways" have proliferated in ways that have reduced each person's unique story to simplistic recipes. More often than not, this cookbook approach ends up telling patients what they *don't* have—which, while potentially reassuring, does not result in a real diagnosis.[1]

Imagine how this approach would work in another setting. Say there is a detective who is trying to solve a murder. He becomes fixated on making sure a certain suspect is *not* the murderer. He spends all of his time ordering surveillance, wire-tapping, and checking the backstory of the first suspect, and it's not until a month later that he's ready to chase down suspects two and three—all the while the real murderer is on the loose and has had more time to wreak havoc undetected. This is not so different from the effects of cookbook medicine, which can lead doctors and patients down the path of unnecessary testing, unwanted anxiety, and, in some cases, real harm because of the delayed diagnosis.

Like many doctors today, Dr. M. is trained to think using **algorithms,** or a **cookbook approach**[2]: if the patient has "chief complaint" A, then ask about risk factors 1, 2, 3. If present, then do a "work up" with tests I, II, III. If negative, then diagnoses x, y, and z can be "ruled out," so consider additional tests IV, V, and VI. And so on and so forth goes the patient through the assembly line. At the end of the day, thousands of dollars of tests can be ordered and months of discomfort endured without ever identifying the **diagnosis,** the disease process, that prompted the symptoms in the first place. Patients can go from the ER to their primary care doctor's office to any number of specialists without ever learning what's really wrong or how they can be made to feel better.

This is **cookbook medicine.** We call it cookbook because it implies there is no deviation from the set **recipe** even as circumstances change. Actually, the term may be unfair to chefs because good chefs would never dream of strictly following their own recipes. Recipes can be helpful as a guideline—but what happens if the asparagus at the market that day is wonderful and fresh, but twice as thick as any asparagus they usually use? Surely, that means they need to adjust their cooking style. Perhaps the asparagus will have to be steamed for twice as long; perhaps this timing will now affect the tempo of the rest of the ingredients; and so on. Cooking solely by recipe produces cafeteria-style meals, a product we'd shy away from eating, much less rely on for our medical care.

Just like cookbook cooking, cookbook medicine is easy to learn and relatively simple to practice.[3] But patients like Jerry end up receiving sub-standard, "cafeteria quality" care. They leave dissatisfied because they came to find out what's wrong and they leave knowing, at best, what they don't have. Doctors end up adopting the role of automaton, following recipes and doing as directed, but no longer empowered to listen, to think, to di-agnose, and to heal. Patients end up believing that their role is to help speed the checkbox ticking as quietly and as obediently as possible. Worse still, they begin to internalize that this is the best and *only* way to receive medical care.

In addition to exacerbating mutual frustration from doctors and pa-tients both, cookbook medicine has contributed to the extraordinary bal-looning of medical care costs. Doctors order more tests not because there is rationale based on the patient in front of them, but because this has become the new "gold" standard in America, the "best" we have to offer. And when prescription pads fill up with tests, patients also demand them, as if tests were cures in and of themselves. It's not difficult to see how the cost of health-care adds up exponentially when doctors and patients both depend on tests, without questioning whether the extra tests are necessary, or worse yet, whether they may be harmful. Everyone gets trapped in an increasingly costly and increasingly dysfunctional system.

There are abundant statistics that describe the skyrocketing cost and declining quality of healthcare. The United States spends close to $2.5 tril-lion on healthcare, over 16 percent of our gross domestic product.[4] Yet, more than 50 million people remain uninsured, and those who are insured are burdened with high costs of healthcare that leave many bankrupt [5] Even though we have the most advanced technologies around the world, the United States consistently ranks below other developed countries in terms of our healthcare system performance.[6] Excessive testing is estimated to contribute $250 billion each year to the overall cost of healthcare.[7] A semi-nal report by the Institute of Medicine found that 100,000 people die of medical error every year in the United States, more than the number that lose their lives to stroke, diabetes, and motor-vehicle accidents combined.[8] Error in diagnosis is by far the largest component of medical error. One in twenty hospitalized patients who die will die because of misdiagnosis, and far more suffer because they never find out their diagnosis.[9]

Attempts to improve the U.S. healthcare system have focused on cost-cutting measures that are often draconian and ineffective. Private insurance companies and public government agencies have tried to rein in costs by limiting treatment options and requiring doctors to follow algorithms around the ordering of tests, with little success to show for it. We believe that forbidding treatments just because they are expensive is not the right approach to healthcare reform. Similarly, reducing medical care to cookbook recipes is not the way to making medicine safer or more efficient.

Too often, healthcare reform targets its efforts toward the medical *industry*. However, medical *practice* centers on the relationship between the individual patient and the individual doctor. This is where reform needs to focus: we need better, leaner, and individualized care for each patient, starting with an accurate diagnosis. There is an urgent need to reform the U.S. healthcare system, but you shouldn't have to wait until then to improve your own healthcare. To the contrary, you can start today, by transforming how you approach your doctor.

Dr. Leana Wen: I've wanted to be a doctor for as long as I can remember. Growing up in China, I had terrible asthma. My earliest memories are of my parents bundling me up in the cold of the winter and shuttling me to hospitals while I gasped for breaths, then putting me on machines to help me breathe. My doctors were so kind to me, and I had this idealist view of what it meant to be a healer.

I am really grateful that I have been able to pursue my childhood dream. In a lot of ways, the process of becoming a doctor has been an incredible journey. In my training, I have learned from brilliant professors and colleagues. At my hospitals, I draw upon the latest technologists and the best specialists to find solutions for my patients. Every day, my job is fulfilling because I am there for my patients in their times of great need.

There was one part of my job, though, that was unsettling. As I proceeded in my training, I began to see that many patients I encountered were being steered onto set diagnostic pathways. Our teachers did it, expounding on "algorithms," which were basically recipes that lumped patients into groups with similar symptoms. Our peers did it, noting how much faster it was to see patients not as Mrs. Smith, the chatty mother of four, or Father Cogliano, the Italian priest, but as their "chief complaints" of headache and abdominal pain.

Without realizing it, this became my practice, too. Patient with chest pain? Follow this **pathway,** appropriately called the "chest pain pathway," because most everyone with chest pain gets the same tests. Abdominal pain? Ask these ten questions and follow the algorithm. Headache? Shortness of breath? Change in mental status? Believe it or not, there are cookbook approaches for all of them. It's supposed to be scientific and based on evidence, so that's good, right? Yet, our patients were leaving confused and unhappy. They felt as if their doctors weren't listening to them, that who they were or why they had come to the doctor didn't matter.

My mother was diagnosed with cancer when I was a medical student. Seeing how she was treated by her providers gave me a whole new understanding of what it meant to be a patient—and why it's so important for both patients and physicians to question this cookbook approach to medicine. I met Josh, and other physicians around the country, who are also fed up with algorithms and recipes. They taught me that there is another approach that is better for patients, incorporating rigorous science along with common sense and the often-forgotten art of medicine. This is the kind medicine that I went to medical school to learn, the kind of medicine that I want my loved ones to receive. This is the kind of care that I want to provide to my patients.

Dr. Josh Kosowsky: I have been practicing medicine for over fifteen years. My father is a doctor, too—a cardiologist. Since the time he went through medical training, medicine has changed almost beyond recognition. When my father was in medical school, he couldn't have dreamed of MRI machines providing high-definition images of the deep recesses of the brain or of patients swallowing tiny pill cameras to take pictures inside the gastrointestinal tract. Now these are commonplace.

Many of these advances have been phenomenal in improving diagnosis. But along with advances in technology, there has been a failure in the way doctors are being trained to think. By this I refer to the "**diagnostic algorithms**," "**rules**," and "**pathways**"—all the components of cookbook medicine.

Don't get me wrong: standardizing medical practice and providing a consistent level of care makes sense. However, by relying on algorithms to the exclusion of everything else, it's as if all patients are meant to be treated exactly the same, simply because they have the same "chief complaint." It just doesn't work.

I've watched a lot of doctors adopt this approach. I'm talking about impressionable young doctors starting their training as well as seasoned senior doctors who are doing the training. Part of my professional responsibility is teaching medical students, and I know that what they hear from me is different from what they're hearing from their other professors. What I try to emphasize to students, even at the earliest stages of their training, is that the key to helping patients is to try and arrive together at a diagnosis. And the key to diagnosis is right in front of us: it lies in our patient and his or her story, not in a recipe that reduces a patient to a symptom or two.

Dr. Wen: This is the concept we aim to teach you: that, as a patient, you can dramatically improve your medical care by focusing on this strikingly simple concept of the diagnosis. If you and your doctor are aiming for a diagnosis from the very start, the attention is focused on you and your story, not just on your symptoms. Instead of forcing you onto a cookie-cutter pathway, your doctor will need to consider each part of your story with you to come up with an answer.

Don't get us wrong; Josh and I aren't saying that we should do away with all attempts to standardize medical care. Our colleague at Brigham and Women's Hospital in Boston, Dr. Atul Gawande, revolutionized the use of simple rules to prevent infections in the intensive care units and operating rooms. Using a checklist to make sure that hands are washed or to verify that operating tools are accounted for is common sense. Likewise, algorithms can play a role in ensuring that doctors have thought of everything before arriving at the diagnosis, like a final mental checklist.

Dr. Kosowsky: Our point is that these rules and algorithms should not be relied upon at the expense of, or to the exclusion of, the individual patient. Each patient's story should be considered on its own terms before deciding how to proceed. That's also just common sense.

We advocate for a transformation in medicine by returning to the fundamental partnership between physician and patient. We teach you that working toward a diagnosis is the one simple concept that will revolutionize your healthcare. The two of us began our crusade for this individualized, leaner, and better approach to medical care by writing articles and lecturing to other physicians, nurses, and public health professionals. Many healthcare providers have joined us, but we quickly learned that there is no point in advocating for change unless we can involve the most important group in this reform: our patients.

That is our hope in writing this book. By telling our stories and those of our patients, we wish to demonstrate the problem with the care you are getting now, how it can be different, and how we can achieve it together. We are driven to teach you—our patients, our readers—how to improve your own care, and by extension, how to improve our healthcare system overall. Our book is not about cutting tests for the sake of reducing cost; it's about getting to the right test and arriving at the right diagnosis. We are not indicting doctors for poor care; we are pointing out a fundamental flaw in the way our healthcare system has evolved and how our doctors are being trained. We are inviting you to become partners in the most important part of your healthcare: your diagnosis. We believe that the key to healthcare reform begins with each patient, and that you can be the one to lead the way.

Since we are both emergency physicians, our stories come from the ER. Probably more so than any other field in medicine, emergency medicine is susceptible to the use (or rather, misuse) of recipes. The fast-moving nature of our work, the breadth of knowledge demanded of practitioners, and the speed and urgency inherent in the patient encounter requires precision and decisiveness. Unfortunately, the solution many ER doctors turn to is to take comfort in algorithms. So millions of dollars of unnecessary lab tests and X-rays and CTs and MRIs are ordered, to the detriment of our healthcare system. And patients end up leaving the ER anemic and irradiated, dissatisfied and frustrated, with no better understanding of what caused their symptoms.

It doesn't have to be this way! If we, as ER doctors, can take the time to talk to our patients and figure out their diagnoses, then every doctor should be able to. If our patients can make themselves heard in the busy and often chaotic setting of the ER, then they can also take these lessons and apply them to their family doctor, their cardiologist, and their diabetes specialist. Our stories may come from the ER, but the lessons we offer are applicable to every doctor, every hospital, and every patient.

Sifting through a patient's story, thinking through the possibilities, and arriving at a diagnosis sounds like the stuff of a good mystery novel. Indeed, the analogy has been made that being a doctor is like being a detective in that both have to sort through clues and be attentive to detail. Our book, though, is not about exotic diagnoses or unusual presentations, but rather about common problems that can be solved better through a partnership between patients and their doctors. We don't talk about flesh-eating bugs from central Africa or one-in-ten-million diseases that ravage obscure neural pathways; we discuss abdominal pain and chest pain; appendicitis and heart attacks; viral syndromes and hangovers.

While we spend some time talking about how doctors think, we don't harp on the successes of the greatest doctors in the world or the horrific failures of the worst doctors. We refer to the everyday doctor, the doctor who will diagnose your sinus infection and the one who will attend to your ailing grandmother in the hospital. We talk about the traps that ordinary patients find themselves in when they go to their doctor with ordinary problems, and we give practical tips for what you can do about it. Our central premise is that doctors are not listening to their patients, leading to misdiagnoses—and often, no diagnosis at all. We propose a model that you can use to guide your doctors to make better diagnoses and to deliver better care. Medicine is urgently in need of change, and we show you how to make a difference in your own healthcare.

Denise Valiant is a thirty-four-year-old woman who lives in Plymouth, New Hampshire. Plymouth is a small town that borders the White Mountain National Forest and is home to Plymouth State University, where Denise is an occasional lecturer in the English department. She spends most of her days at home, raising her seven-year-old twin sons and occasionally working on her book, a collection of short stories.

One day, Denise found herself far from Plymouth. She had just been through a hair-raising two-and-a-half-hour ambulance ride, and now she was in Boston, Massachusetts, sitting on a stretcher in the ER.

When she woke up that morning, she could not have anticipated that she would be going so far from Plymouth. She hadn't felt right the night before, and that morning, she began vomiting and having diarrhea. She wasn't keeping down any food, and her sister urged her to go to the local ER to get checked out. Her husband was out of town for business, so she dropped her kids off with her sister and went to the ER.

In the ER, she had an IV placed and some blood drawn. A nurse and then a doctor asked her a few questions. Before she knew it, she was drinking some foul-smelling liquid. It was for a CT scan, she was told, though nobody had mentioned to her that she was getting a CT. They must know what they are doing, she thought, so she dutifully drank the liquid, and a couple of hours later, she went into a donut-shaped machine.

It took another couple of hours to hear about the results. In the meantime, Denise was actually feeling better. She wasn't particularly nauseous, and she even felt hungry. Her sister called—she had developed similar symptoms, and so did her daughter. On the phone, she could tell that her twins were getting rowdy and wanted to go home. Denise was tired and wanted to go home, too.

Soon, she got the news. The CT scan found something concerning. It looked like maybe there was a mass in her pancreas. A mass-like cancer? How could that be? The first doctor came in and told her that this could be an emergency. They were going to send her to one of the area's top hospitals, in Boston, to figure out what to do next.

Denise was scared. She didn't want to go all the way to Boston. She felt better, but everyone was telling her that her life could be in danger. Something must be terribly wrong.

So that was how Denise from Plymouth, New Hampshire, ended up 120 miles away from home. By the time she arrived in Boston, it had been ten hours after she first went to the ER in her hometown. More people came to take her details. She got more blood drawn. She saw a new set of doctors and nurses. They poked her belly. "Ow!" she said when someone who said he was a surgeon pressed on her particularly hard. He looked concerned. There were whispers and a few nods. She didn't understand—

was she getting surgery? Nobody was giving her a straight answer. They had to discuss it more, they said. She was told that the CT scan she had done in New Hampshire was "insufficient" and they would have to do another one. She drank more smelly liquid. She waited. She got into another donut-shaped machine.

Eventually, they came in to tell her the good news: the CT scan was normal after all. It seems there was no mass in her pancreas; actually, her pancreas looked fine. She didn't have appendicitis. (Of course not! She had her appendix out as a kid!) She probably had food poisoning or a viral illness. Well, she could have told them that hours ago, back in Plymouth! But now, she was a hundred miles away from home, with no way to get back. Her sister was with all the kids and wasn't about to drive two hours each way—especially since it was after midnight. She would need to get a cab, or pay for a hotel until someone could pick her up in the morning.

Nevertheless, she was OK. She should be thankful for that. She was feeling better; she didn't have cancer or need surgery; there was nothing wrong. Yes, this was all good! She gathered her belongings and thanked her doctors.

But this had not been a good day at all.

Dr. Kosowsky: I was working that night in the ER when Denise came in. She wasn't my patient, but I heard another doctor talk about the unfortunate woman who was sent all the way from New Hampshire to hear that the CT result that was supposedly abnormal wasn't abnormal at all. The story itself wasn't at all uncommon; believe it or not, we see a lot of cases like Denise's. What I found fascinating was my colleague's conclusion.

"That hospital needs to get a better CT scanner," she said.

A resident overhearing this conversation commented that they should get a better radiologist who could read the scans right. A nurse asked why they couldn't just do a repeat CT themselves instead of transferring her to us. Nobody asked what I thought was the critical question: why did she even get a CT in the first place? This was a young, healthy woman with stomach flu. Why did she even get blood drawn, except that it was a reflex reaction for everyone with abdominal pain? If the initial doctor had taken a better history aimed at figuring out her diagnosis, he would have concluded this, too, and Denise could have avoided the entire escalation of care that ended up with her getting not one, but *two* CTs in one day and her being transported a hundred of miles away from home.

Dr. Wen: This story had a relatively happy ending: Denise eventually arrived home, felt better, and moved on with her life. When we interviewed her, she told us all about how thankful she is that she had such good doctors. I'm glad she has such an optimistic approach to the situation, but, like Josh, I don't think her doctors were all that good! This is a patient who got quite a few unnecessary tests, starting with the first unnecessary CT that then triggered this whole other chain of events.

Dr. Kosowsky: Think about how different Denise's case would have been if that very first doctor had listened to her story. Not just asked her a list of questions, but really listened to how her symptoms started and what they were like.

Dr. Wen: And how different would things have been if she were involved in the decision-making? If she had known to ask questions such as, "What are we looking for on this test? What are the alternatives?" And most important, "What diagnosis are we working toward?"

A few months ago, we attended a dinner with a group of friends, all nonmedical professionals. There were a couple of lawyers, a math teacher, a university vice-chancellor, a public relations consultant, a writer, and an engineer. We told them about the principles behind this book and the concept of individualized medical care and the importance of diagnosis.

The reception was unanimously positive. "Of course," everyone said. "That's the way medical care should be; it's common sense."

Yet, the same ideas when presented to a group of doctors are met with skepticism at best and cynical laughter at worst. It's too naïve, too idealistic, these doctors say. It may sound good in theory, but it's just not possible. What hope is there when medical students are taught more and more about rules and recipes, and proportionately less about listening to patients and making diagnoses? What can this book do in the face of doctors getting paid to do more tests rather than less, and the reimbursement structure not allowing time for history-taking? Even the cost-cutting practices by insurance companies result in more algorithms and less thinking. And patients, too—aren't they the ones demanding the newest scans and tests that they see on TV? Won't they sue their doctor if they don't get them?

The cynics are wrong, because we know that our patients are on our side. The real beneficiaries and the primary stakeholders of the medical practice are the patients. At the end of the day, patients have the right (as long as they are aware of it) to demand the best care possible, even if that means changing physicians. Cynicism should be contained to hopeless situations where no workable solution is imaginable. However, neither doctors nor patients need to work hard to imagine what alternatives to cookbook medicine might be, because we practiced them not so long ago.

What's more is that we don't need years of research to come up with answers: the ideas that seem so foreign to most doctors indoctrinated into a dysfunctional system are very much intuitive to everyone else. Our patients don't go to the doctor so that they can be told what recipe they fall under. They don't go because they want unnecessary tests that result in increased personal financial pressure and worsening burden to our already-taxed healthcare systems. They don't go because they want long hospital stays and large doses of radiation. Rather, our patients go the doctor to find out quickly, inexpensively, and compassionately what they have. They want their doctors to listen to them and think through decisions together. Ultimately, they want to feel better.

It's to guide our patients in their next healthcare encounters that we write this book. It's to show you how medical care *ought* to be that we ask you for your partnership. In the process of illustrating what's wrong with our system of care and how we can improve it, we are signaling your importance in this task, and how it will only truly be accomplished through a partnership between doctor and patient. Whether you or a loved one has received disappointing or stellar care, or will in the years to come, this book will help you ensure that you get the medical care you deserve.

When Doctors Don't Listen uses a combination of patient stories and our two perspectives and experiences as practicing ER physicians to help you understand what is happening with your medical care and you how you can improve it. Every patient story is based on what we have witnessed personally and on interviews with the individuals involved. Our patients wished for us to tell their stories, but because of the sensitive nature of the information disclosed, we have changed names and identifying characteristics and used composite characters in some instances. We also include interviews with physicians; their names are actual names unless otherwise specified.

In between the stories, we present our interpretations and lessons. You will notice that we write either as a collective voice (what you are reading right now), or using our individual voices (these are preceded by our names). The separate narratives are used to illustrate our two perspectives, as physician-in-training and as senior physician.

Our book is divided into five sections. The first part explores how we got to the point of accepting cookbook medicine. The second part illustrates the pitfalls of cookbook medicine with four cases from the ER and the downstream implications for patients, doctors, and the healthcare system. We demonstrate how things can be different in the third and fourth sections, which describe the fundamentals of an active patient-doctor partnership and how these apply to real-life scenarios with The 8 Pillars to Better Diagnosis and Prescriptions for Patients. We discuss how they can be applied, with vastly different outcomes, to the four cases in Part II. The fifth and final section examines the larger implications of this approach to healthcare policy and reform.

This is a practical book. Every chapter is replete with tips. Look out for 911 Action Tips interspersed in the text when you see this symbol: ✚. These highlight the most relevant tips as you can apply them to your doctor: when and how you should ask questions and which questions yield the most important answers. Each chapter ends with 911 Review, a summary of key take-home points. There are additional exercises and worksheets to assist you and allow you to practice what you read.

This is not a conventional book. It may not be an easy read. If you are a healthcare provider, it could challenge the way that you practice medicine and see your patients. If you are a patient, it could change the way you think about your doctors and interact with them. As you read this book, we hope that you consider challenging conventional wisdom and asking with us whether there is a better way. We aim for this to be the opening salvo of a revolution among patients to improve the quality of their own care and to lead the way to true healthcare reform. We hope you will strive with us to advance the goal of better diagnosis and better medical care.

911 REVIEW

- Cookbook recipes, "algorithms," "pathways," and "formulas" lead to inaccurate diagnoses, astronomical healthcare costs, and unhappy patients.
- This book provides practical tips for you to advocate for your health—starting with a simple yet critical component of your care: your diagnosis.
- Advocating for your health is the first step toward meaningful healthcare reform.

Part I

How We Got Here

Cookbook medicine did not come into being overnight. To understand how we have come to accept the widespread use of recipes and algorithms, we begin with a brief history of medical diagnosis. In Chapter 1, we discuss the Four Eras of Diagnosis: how medical diagnosis has evolved, or perhaps devolved, over time. In Chapter 2, we describe the training of physicians and how this fosters cookbook medicine.

One

From Shamans to Black Boxes

Arthur Coates is a partner in one of Boston's most prestigious law firms. At fifty-seven, with more than thirty years of malpractice law under his belt, Arthur is known in the business as being "sharp as a tack, with the instinct of a killer whale." Today was the culmination of a multibillion-dollar lawsuit involving a local hospital and several of its staff. It was just before lunchtime, and he was cross-examining the last witness when a most remarkable incident occurred.

"Were you aware that my client had a previous history of heart disease?" Arthur asked the witness. He was pacing the room with a steady, deliberate gait, a style characteristic for him, noted his younger colleague, Tim Simcock, who was watching from gallery.

As the witness was about to respond, Arthur spoke again, this time appearing to direct the question to the judge.

"Were you aware of my client's previous history of heart disease?" he asked.

What a strange strategy to repeat the question like that? Tim thought. Maybe this is how Arthur does things; perhaps Tim should take notes on Arthur's style. The opposing attorney objected, but the judge motioned to the witness to answer anyway.

"I don't recall," he stated.

"Did you know about my client's heart disease?" Arthur asked again, this time to no one in particular. "Were you aware that my client had suffered previously from heart disease?"

The opposing attorney got on his feet, yelling, "Objection—asked and answered!" but Arthur went on asking the same question several more times. Tim saw that Arthur's gait had sped up. It wasn't unsteady, but he wasn't walking in any particular direction. Could it be that the great Arthur Coates couldn't remember what else he had to ask? Tim stood up to approach the bench and request a sidebar. As he got closer, he saw that beads of sweat were pouring down Arthur's face. The judge was banging his gavel, but Arthur appeared to take no notice. The entire room was watching Arthur, transfixed. There were murmurs. What's happening? Is it a trick? Is Arthur Coates having a breakdown?

"There is something wrong!" Tim shouted. "He needs a doctor!"

A recess was called. As it happens, there *was* a doctor in the courtroom—the one who Arthur had just been questioning. The doctor stepped from the witness box and cautiously made his way over to his former interrogator, who was now crouched in the middle of the courtroom like a vanquished gladiator, his head buried in his hands.

"Are you OK? Do you need help?" In a curious reversal of roles, it was the doctor asking the questions.

Arthur shook his head. "Do I know you?"

How bizarre! This was one of the most sought-after minds in his profession, and he couldn't remember a key witness? But not only couldn't Arthur recall any details of the case, he didn't know that he was in court or that the year was 2012.

"I think he may be having a stroke," concluded the doctor, a gynecologist by training, but familiar enough with basic neurology to know that sudden memory loss was potentially quite serious. "Someone call for an ambulance!"

"Who are you again?" Arthur asked Tim quizzically as they rode together in the back of the ambulance.

Tim sighed. It was the third time Arthur had asked him this question since leaving the courthouse. "Tim. We've worked at the same firm for the past eight years. We golf together. Our wives are in the same book club."

"Oh," Arthur replied. To Tim, it looked as if his colleague registered what he just said, but a few minutes later, when he asked Arthur if he remembered him, Arthur shrugged. He was apologetic, but really—he just didn't remember.

This was how Arthur Coates presented to us in the ER. On the surface, Arthur appeared like any other high-powered lawyer: middle-aged, distinguished-looking, with a dark power suit and blood-red tie. He feels great, he said. And yet he had no clue what day of the week or what month it was. He nodded when he's told that he's at a hospital in Boston, but a few minutes later, he no longer remembered this. When he was asked to recall three objects—a pencil, a lamp, and a curtain—he could repeat them back instantaneously, but a minute later, he could not remember any of them. Interestingly, though, he knew that he was born in 1953 in Omaha, Nebraska. He told us that his childhood best friend was a scrawny kid named Auggie and that his first dog was a yippy tan Yorkshire terrier.

The rest of Arthur's history and physical exam was unremarkable. His wife, Amy, arrived and confirmed that Arthur was generally healthy. He'd never had anything like this happen before. In fact, he hadn't missed a day of work in his life. He took no medications other than a baby aspirin each morning, and he went to the gym three times a week. He hadn't been traveling to any exotic locations, and nobody around him had been sick. His vital signs were all normal, as was his vision, hearing, speech, and gross motor and sensory function. He had normal reflexes, coordination, balance, and gait. When asked to perform basic addition and subtraction or spell "W-O-R-L-D" backward, he seemed to have no difficulty whatsoever.

Could the great Arthur Coates have had a nervous breakdown? Tim wondered. It had been a stressful few weeks leading up to the trial, and this morning's proceedings had more than their share of tense moments. "But this is a guy who's argued dozens of cases like this! It's just not like him to react this way!"

Arthur's behavior may seem bizarre, but he was actually exhibiting classic signs of a disease called "transient global ischemia." First described in the 1970s in a case involving a farmer who drove a tractor onto a busy highway because he could not remember who he was or where he was going,[1] transient global ischemia is characterized by a sudden loss of recent memory. Patients tend to recall deeply encoded, distant events like childhood memories, but not recent happenings. Other than memory failure, they do not have any other neurological deficits. The cause of this ailment is unknown, though it is more common in males than females, and there is some association with a prior stressful or emotional event. The symptoms are self-resolving, usually completely disappearing within twenty-four hours.

Because transient global ischemia is so highly classic and specific, afflicted patients can be sent home to await symptom resolution as long as the caretakers at home are comfortable taking care of them. Twenty years ago, Arthur could have been diagnosed based on his clinical presentation alone. No further workup would have been provided, because it was clear what he had. Today, even though his diagnosis could have been made just by hearing his story, the doctors taking care of Arthur were petrified of him going home to recover on his own. Our discussion in the ER went like this: what if we were missing something bad, something really bad? What if he was having some type of stroke that we hadn't thought of? Some unusual metabolic disease?

Never mind that Arthur exhibited none of the signs concerning for this smorgasbord of bad diseases. Yet, the resulting management was predictable: to be "on the safe side," Arthur was told he needed to go through the entire battery of tests. So he got a head CT to make sure he didn't have bleeding in his brain. His CT was normal, so an MRI was ordered to look for a more subtle stroke. In the meantime, his blood tests, chest X-ray, and EKG also came back normal and offered no explanation for his symptoms, so the neurologists were called to see Arthur. After several hours of consultation, and with absolutely normal tests, their conclusions were similar to ours: "Symptoms are consistent with transient global ischemia," they wrote, "but we cannot exclude transient thromboembolic phenomenon or atypical seizure activity." They recommended further studies to "rule out" these remote possibilities, not acknowledging the difficulty of proving a negative.

So Arthur waited in the hospital overnight. By later that evening, he was pretty much back to normal. But there were still more tests to do. Arthur stayed overnight to have brain wave tests to make sure he was not having a seizure (he wasn't) and an ultrasound of his heart to confirm that his heart valves were normal (they were). Finally, late the next evening, he was discharged home, some thirty-six hours after Tim and the ambulance crew brought him in.

Why is it that Arthur Coates stayed in the hospital at a cost of tens of thousands of dollars in studies, procedures, and specialists' time, when he could have been sent home in the first place? Why did we need blood draws and radiation to conclude that he didn't have diseases that he never showed signs of? Why couldn't doctors have provided the reassurance of both the diagnosis and the expected course of his illness, sparing him and his family many fretful hours worrying about heart attacks and strokes and seizures and whether they would ever have the old Arthur Coates back?

We were there—we can tell you why. It's because doctors today no longer think that patients can be relied upon to tell the history of their illness. It's because "ruling out" bad diseases has taken precedence over making a diagnosis. It's because we have elaborate tests available at our fingertips, and both doctors and patients have an unshakable belief in technology. Never mind that the fancy tests add little value, especially when used to exclude diagnoses that weren't likely in the first place.[2] Never mind that the procedures may actually impose risk or cause actual harm.

Diseases have always existed, but modern technology has not always been available. To explain how far we have come, for better and for worse, we present a brief history of medical diagnosis. We identify four periods, what we term the Four Eras of Diagnosis. As you read, think about the three patients you've been introduced to: Jerry the mechanic with chest tightness, Denise the housewife with vomiting and diarrhea, and Arthur the lawyer with sudden memory loss. How would the diagnostic process been different in each of the four eras? Would their care have been better then or now? Would yours?

Let's call the First Era of Diagnosis the "Era of Spiritual Healing and Magical Thinking." Records dating back thousands of years have described shamans, faith healers, and their equivalents as healers who provided what would now be called medical care through spiritual means. Virtually every ancient society had one such person or a designated group of people who was said to possess the magical powers to heal—and as a prerequisite to that, to diagnose.[3]

Many of these ancient faith healers had knowledge of local plants and herbs and made liberal use of medicinal concoctions in their practice. Others utilized the power of chants and group prayer. The Peruvian Amazons believed that spirits would teach their shaman, the "curandero," a song; the shaman's job was to learn the song in order to figure out the specific illness.[4] In other cultures, the key to diagnosis lay in the identification of the appropriate evil spirit, and the faith healer's job was to possess the body of the ill and chase out the spirit causing harm. In the Hmong culture, the healer, called the "Shi Yi," was said to restore health by calling the soul of the sick from travels with bad spirits and back into the human body.[5]

This form of healing, grounded in belief of spirits and magic, seems worlds apart from medicine as we know it today. But there is something of this First Era that we still find in modern medicine: the notion of implicit trust. Then, as now, those who are sick entrust their health and well-being to a designated healer. In ancient times, illness was a literal black box: you tell your healer your problems, the healer shakes a black box, and out comes a solution of some kind. As a faithful member of the community, you trust your healer and accept the outcome.

Why do we even mention this era when we can take it at face value that few of us would prefer to live back in the land of shamans and black boxes? We discuss it because this era is not entirely in the past. Alternative healing methods are actively practiced today. Many societies continue to rely on shamans and faith healers. In the United States, 74 percent of patients report that they use complementary and alternative therapies in addition to Western medicine, including herbs and "new age" medicine techniques such as *qi gong* spiritual healing and *reiki* energy healing.[6]

It's interesting to note that these alternative healing modalities continue to emphasize the patient first and foremost. Making a diagnosis requires attention to the individual and his stories. In addition, because healers are typically from the same community as their patients, cultural context is necessarily taken into account as part of the diagnostic process. In all cases, a diagnosis (whether correct or not) is given, with treatment tailored to fix the problem identified. Perhaps as a result, these forms of treatment result in total commitment from the patient and their families, and adherence to the treatment regimen tends to be very high.

With the dawn of recorded history came the Second Era of Diagnosis, which we call the "Era of Early Empiricism and Disease Classification." As far back as 2000 B.C., the Egyptian scholar Imhotep wrote the medical textbook known as the *Edwin Smith Papyrus*.[7] This is the first known text in the ancient world to describe in detail a method of diagnosis whereby each disease has corresponding symptoms and physical findings.[8] A subsequent Babylonian text, *The Diagnostic Handbook,* introduced the role of empiricism and logic in diagnosis, focusing on rules for predicting when and how a constellation of symptoms and signs represented a particular disease state.[9]

The Father of Western Medicine, Hippocrates, was the preeminent physician of his time, and his works epitomize the diagnostic approach in this Second Era. Hippocrates was deeply invested in describing the **natural history of illnesses**—how symptoms came together and how they progressed over time. For example, he was one of the first to describe epilepsy as a syndrome of uncontrolled, recurrent seizures. It was not known what caused it or how to prevent the seizures from recurring (many contemporaries continued to believe that they were a form of "possession" by evil spirits), but Hippocrates noted that lying the patient flat on the ground was beneficial (at the very least, to prevent the patients from further injuring himself or others). Hippocrates also recognized the syndrome of persistent cough, fever, and wasting as pneumonia, which he described as a contagious disease because family members and close contacts appeared to contract it. Unfortunately, this was often a fatal diagnosis, as there was no cure at the time.

Though Hippocrates's focus was on disease description and not on diagnosis per se,[10] his detailed writings allowed for progress. Patterns of symptoms formed the basis of disease classification, and pattern recognition became the basis of diagnosis and medical reasoning. In Hippocrates's time, few other diagnostic tools existed; moreover, the ancient Greek taboo against dissection meant that little was known about the anatomical basis of disease. Under the tutelage of a master physician, students would learn to recognize common illnesses by learning about and then observing patterns of signs and symptoms. Over time, new diseases would be described and their natural histories recounted. Physicians practicing in this Second Era relied almost exclusively on interactions with their patients and their families, not dissimilar to the First Era.

It was during Hippocrates's time that the idea of the "expert physician" first emerged. Hippocrates himself was regarded as one, along with several of his contemporaries. These were physicians that patients traveled to from near and far to get their expert opinion, and students huddled in amphitheaters into the wee hours to listen to their ruminations. Even at this early juncture, medicine was coming to be recognized as a **practice**—a process of learning that takes years to refine and perfect.

Fast-forward a couple of thousands years. Advances in anatomy, physiology, and other sciences during the eighteenth and nineteenth centuries paved the way to the Third Era of Diagnosis: the Golden Age of Medical Diagnosis, in which both the science and art of medicine reached new heights. By the 1800s, enough was understood about the scientific basis of disease that diagnosis became more than pattern recognition; it also involved understanding mechanisms of disease and how the disease could be prevented and treated. Diagnosis was no longer simply based on ritual, be it the shaman's black box or the classical physician's systems of classification. Doctors could now not only make sense of the natural history of disease, but also then potentially modify it.

Despite the burgeoning scientific advances, this Third Era was still noted for its emphasis on the art of diagnosis. There was no more prominent figure in this era than Sir William Osler. Born in 1849, Sir William was one of the founding professors at Johns Hopkins Hospital and the first professor of medicine there. Osler taught his students that the best textbook of medicine was the patient himself. Before applying any tests, obtaining a complete and accurate account of the history from the patient was paramount. Osler's belief in the importance of the patient-doctor relationship led him to pioneer significant reforms in medical education, reducing the classroom time to allow students to devote a larger proportion of their time to direct interaction with patients.[11]

In the Golden Age of Medical Diagnosis, the interplay of the "art" and "science" was exemplified in the daily practice of the country family doctor, the general practitioner (G.P.). The G.P. took pride in knowing each member of the town, in being present for the delivery of every child, in giving the child's every vaccination and treating every broken bone, and in delivering, in years to come, the child's child. The G.P. made home visits and understood the context of his patients' illness in the most literal sense. The doctor had training in the scientific underpinnings of disease and had few additional tools (like a stethoscope, perhaps, or some simple blood or urine tests) at his disposal, but the emphasis was on the patient's story, with an equal mix of medical knowledge and common sense helping to forge the indelible bond between the doctor and patient.

It is this era of medicine to which many doctors and patients now look with nostalgia. Older doctors frequently bemoan the fading emphasis on the art of medicine, and those who practiced in the waning days of the Golden Age speak of the time spent listening to their patients, of developing an intimate familiarity not only with their patients' individual histories, but also with how the disease affects each particular patient. When they went to their G.P., patients were confident that someone who cared about them was listening to their story and doing his best to diagnose and to heal.

If this Golden Era was so great, then what happened to it? Are we really advocating for a return to the way things used to be some fifty or one hundred years ago?

In many ways, science and technology have brought positive impact on medical practice. Heart attacks used to be untreatable. Now, little wires can snake through vessels in the groin to open up blockages and restore blood flow to the heart. Abdominal surgery used to involve huge scars and weeks and months of recovery time. Now, gallbladder and appendix surgeries are outpatient, same-day procedures. Few would question that scientific and technological advances have revolutionized the *treatment* of diseases.

However, whether science and technology have contributed positively to *diagnosis* is more nuanced. Take the advent of the so-called "evidence-based" algorithms for diagnosis. Instead of carefully listening to a patient and figuring out what disease she has, a doctor can use a recipe to plug symptoms into a formula and come up with a number that represents the likelihood that she *doesn't* have a blood clot or a heart attack. There may be a role for algorithms as a point of reference, but increasingly, physicians will use

these as a substitute to spending time listening to patients and as justification for why a diagnosis is not being made.

Related to this is the increasing reliance on the diagnostic testing. There
is no doubt that blood tests and advanced imaging can reveal much-needed
information. However, tests are not perfect; they can be time-consuming,
not to mention expensive, and every test (even a blood-draw) conveys some
risk. As we discuss in later chapters, tests may also be deceptive in that a
"negative" result may provide false reassurance (and a "positive" may result
in needless anxiety). And tests themselves often become a proxy for decision-
making, with resulting increased cost for the patient and for society. The
irony is that since tests only show what the disease is not, the diagnosis will
still be as much of a mystery as it was to start with.

The reliance on science is not solely to blame for this move away from
the Golden Era of Medical Diagnosis. For one thing, medicine has become
increasingly fragmented; the idea of having "your" doctor is increasingly
becoming a relic of the past. Family doctors and general internists are quick
to refer any condition out of their comfort zone to specialists. Many patients
don't have a choice of a primary care doctor—they are assigned to someone
on the basis of their insurance coverage and the availability of a doctor to
accept new patients. If a change in employment leads to a change in insurance, then tough luck. Our country is facing a critical shortage of physicians,
in particular primary care physicians,[12] and making an appointment with a
new doctor can take weeks to months.

Even having a primary care provider is a luxury. For the one in four
working Americans who don't have health insurance, the only option for
medical care may be the ER or a neighborhood clinic, where invariably
they see a different doctor each time who doesn't know their basic medical
history, let alone who they are as a person.[13] Some would argue that the role
of the ER doctor is simply to "rule out" the worst things that a patient could
have; after all, they are seeking emergency care. We would argue that this
shouldn't be the case; for many of our patients, the ER is their one shot at
healthcare, and they need to get their diagnosis right. If the system of care
does not support this, then patients will get ushered out after a quick "rule-
out" only to return with the same (or worse) symptoms of their undiagnosed
disease.

We cannot discuss the problems with medical care today without mentioning the rise of medical malpractice and its impact on how doctors make decisions.[14] The fear of being sued is real and not at all insignificant: the average ER doctor in the United States is sued once every six years, and pretty much every doctor in every specialty can be expected to be sued in his or her professional lifetime.[15] All doctors know of someone—a supervisor, a colleague, a trainee—who is undergoing what's known euphemistically as an "adverse action." To be sure, there is a small minority of doctors out there who are actually providing substandard care. However, for the vast majority of doctors who are well trained and just doing their best, the medical malpractice system is like a game of Russian roulette: stay in the game long enough, have a patient who ends up with a bad outcome, and your number will come up. So doctors learn to order tests just to be sure that they are "covered." Just in case. Instead of focusing on getting the diagnosis right, doctors consider every conceivable life-threatening diagnosis, however improbable, and feel compelled to "rule out" all of them.

At a certain point, this kind of defensive medicine becomes so pervasive as to define, in a perversely self-fulfilling way, a standard of care in which everyone in the field is overtesting and underdiagnosing. Practiced over and over by physicians across the country, defensive medicine leads to millions of unnecessary tests, escalating the cost of care and further burdening our already-taxed healthcare budget. More insidiously, today's doctors, whose entire training has been in this environment, no longer retain a sense of proportion in considering a patient's presentation. Instead of partnering with the patient to come up with a diagnosis that is the most likely, doctors profess servile adherence to rules and recipes that they believe will protect them from malpractice lawyers.[16] Fear of missing a serious diagnosis, however improbable, dominates medical decision-making to the exclusion of common sense and the patient's best interest.

But it's not just doctors that are to blame; there are expectations that originate from the patient side as well. The consumer movement in healthcare that was initially intended to empower patients has paradoxically led to less involvement in the most important aspect of their care. Certain aspects of the consumer movement have been positive—for example, the increased education of patients on preventive health and shared decision-making in weighing treatment options.[17] On the other hand, in an era of commodified healthcare, the emphasis on consumerism encourages patients to request "the latest and greatest" technologies: screening tests, subspecialty consultations, whole-body MRIs. Rather than empowering patients to engage in the diagnostic process together with their doctors, this movement only further encourages doctors to forgo the traditional patient-doctor relationship and simply order the latest test, resulting paradoxically, in formulaic, depersonalized care.

Taken together, a blind devotion to science and technology, an increasingly dysfunctional healthcare system, and perverse personal and economic incentives have forced a change in the practice of medicine and ushered us into this Fourth Era, the "Era of Depersonalized Diagnosis." It is this aspect of modern medicine that we wish to challenge.

In this Era of Depersonalized Diagnosis, we seem to have come full-circle, back to the time of the black box, when a visit to the shaman turns up a solution in the form of a random incantation or ritual. Today, doctors order a CT or MRI and expect the patient to emerge from the (literal and figurative) black box with an answer. Today, doctors enter disparate pieces of data into a formula and expect it to magically churn out an answer. Why not? It's "safe." It's "standard of practice." It "saves times." It "decreases (or so doctors choose to believe) the risk of malpractice." There's no thinking necessary. But at what cost to patients?

It would be ludicrous to suggest that any of us would rather live in the First Era of shamans or the Second Era under the auspices of ancient Greeks. Most of us would probably not elect to live in the Third Era when the art of healing prevailed, because in today's modern world we do have the luxury of far more sophisticated testing and treatment at our disposal. But perhaps there are elements of the diagnostic art from the previous three eras that have been too hastily discarded. Consider the patients we've met. In a previous era, mechanic Jerry might have been told he had muscle spasms and been sent home with a heating pad; housewife Denise might have been diagnosed with stomach upset and told to drink lots of fluids. Neither would have been burdened with excessive diagnostic tests and wasted thousands of dollars of their money (and ours) only to worry more about what they might have.

Arthur Coates, too, would have gone home, he and his family reassured by the history and physical exam alone that he didn't have a stroke and that he would get better without intervention. He would have received not only less expensive but better, more personalized medical care. Perhaps Arthur can be a lesson to us that there may be aspects of how medicine was practiced in times before that we can learn from today—such as the art of healing and the paramount importance of the diagnosis.

911 REVIEW

- There are lessons to be learned from the past Eras of Diagnosis, such as the importance of making a diagnosis and primacy of the patient-doctor relationship.
- The current Era of Depersonalized Diagnosis has significant advantages over past eras, but also many problems.
- These problems are rooted in our unshakable belief in science, our dysfunctional healthcare system, and the lack of attention to the individual patient.

Two

Do As I Say; Do As I Do

In 1866, a boy named Abraham was born in Louisville, Kentucky, to an immigrant Jewish couple, Moritz and Esther Flexner.[1] The sixth of nine children, Abraham excelled academically, matriculating into Johns Hopkins University in 1884, eight years after the university opened its doors. Moritz's hat business suffered during the depression of the late 1800s, and rather than abandoning his studies, Abraham used his studiousness to graduate in just two years, at the age of nineteen.

Abraham was particularly interested in education,[2] and upon graduation, he returned to his hometown to teach at the public high school. He married a former pupil, Anne Crawford, who went on to have a successful career as a Broadway playwright. In 1890, with Anne's encouragement, Abraham opened a private college preparatory school to test his novel ideas, and wrote a book, *The American College,* that contained a searing account of the failures of higher education. His early successes attracted the attention of Henry Pritchett, the newly appointed president of the Carnegie Foundation, who had been tasked with finding someone to pioneer a study on the problems with American medical training.

The closest Abraham had been to a medical school was through his brother, Simon, a physician who became pathology professor at the University of Louisville.[3] Nevertheless, in 1908, Pritchett selected him to head the study on reforming medical education. Over the next two years, Abraham traversed the United States by horse, train, and buggy to visit all 155 medical schools in existence. In 1910, he published the "Flexner Report," the sentinel study on medical education that revolutionized not only the training of medical doctors in the United States, but also the practice of medicine throughout the world.

We are writing this book one hundred years after Abraham Flexner issued his dictum. In the last chapter, we saw how medical diagnosis has evolved to the current Era of Depersonalized Diagnosis. Now, we examine how the process of medical training itself conspires to take the best and the brightest and dissuade them from the art of diagnosis. How is it that doctors-in-training go from empathic, caring individuals to physicians reliant on algorithms and recipes rather than the patients in front of them? What is it about modern medical training that perpetuates cookbook thinking? Is there any hope for change?

In this chapter, we answer these questions by chronicling how young doctors are trained. First, we explain the steps to becoming a doctor: from medical student, to intern, to resident, and to attending physician. Then, building upon the story of Abraham Flexner, we trace how medical education has changed over the last hundred years. We illustrate how the reforms that started with Flexner have had some unintentional consequences, de-emphasizing diagnosis and diminishing the importance of the doctor-patient relationship. Along the way, we offer our two perspectives: one as supervising physician who went through medical training in the '80s and '90s, and the other as a young doctor who started medical training in the early 2000s and is completing the process now.

"My name is Dr. John Stephens. I'm one of the residents."
"Hi, I'm Alan Jones, the student doctor."
"Ma'am? Hi, I'm the oncology fellow, Nathan Chen."
"I'm Dr. Shah, the attending."

Over the course of a single visit to any major medical center, a patient will encounter multiple doctors in various stages of their training and practice. The titles and descriptors may seem confusing. We give you a quick guide to medical training so that the next time you go to the hospital, you will know where your doctor is in the process of their training and what you can expect from him or her.

Medical training in the United States is, as most of us know, a long and prescribed process.[4] Since almost all medical schools require a bachelor's degree,[5] future doctors must first complete four years of undergraduate work at a college or university. It is not compulsory for these "premedical" students to major in the sciences, but they must take a core of prerequisite science classes such as biology, chemistry, and physics, and score well on the Medical College Admissions Test (MCAT). Getting into medical school is competitive, with a ratio of one matriculant to every three applicants. Most premedical students try to supplement their grades and MCAT scores with time spent in research labs, volunteer experience in hospitals, or other extracurricular service activities.

Once the premed becomes a **medical student,** there are four more years of formal education. There are over 160 allopathic and osteopathic medical schools in the United States today.[6] Most medical schools divide the four years such that the first two years (the "preclinical years") are primarily classroom- and laboratory-based, and the second two years (the "clinical years") involve hands-on clinical training with rotations through the fundamental specialties such as internal medicine, surgery, pediatrics, family medicine, obstetrics-gynecology, emergency medicine, neurology, and psychiatry. Students in their clinical years spend their days in clinics and on hospital wards, working under the supervision of doctors. They are the ones who introduce themselves as "medical student" or "student doctor," and often, they are the first ones to see a patient. Everything they do must be closely supervised by someone else: they can interview patients and suggest diagnoses and treatments, but medical students do not make final treatment decisions or perform procedures by themselves.

All medical schools are affiliated with one or more teaching hospitals, also known as academic medical centers. Harvard Medical School, where we work, is affiliated with Brigham and Women's Hospital, Massachusetts General Hospital, and Boston Children's Hospital, among other hospitals. These teaching hospitals are the training sites of medical students and residents; they also tend to be the hub of pioneering research activity and where the noted specialists practice. From the patient's perspective, teaching hospitals have a trade-off: in exchange for access to the latest medical advances and the best-known specialist in their fields, patients offer to have physicians-in-training learn from them. In many underserved areas, academic medical centers are the main institutions providing charity care, often in ERs that are required by law to see every patient.[7]

On the day they graduate from medical school, the student becomes a medical doctor, an "M.D." but this M.D. alone does not entitle one to practice medicine; in the United States, a new graduate must enter postgraduate training called residency in order to be a licensed physician.[8] During their final year of medical school, students choose a field of specialization and, upon graduation, they enter **residency** training in that field. Residency ranges from three to seven years, depending on the specialty. Internal medicine, pediatrics, and family medicine are three-year residencies. Radiology and ophthalmology are four-year residencies. Emergency medicine can be three or four. General surgery and neurosurgery involve five to seven years of postgraduate training. After completing residency, one is eligible to sit for additional exams (written and/or oral), to qualify as "Board Certified" in a particular specialty.

The three-to-seven years of residency are fabled to be some of the most intensive experiences among all types of professional training. Residency training is predicated on the concept of complete immersion: the term *resident* originated in the early 1900s when new medical school graduates were expected to live in the hospitals throughout their term of service. These residents were expected to live a monastic lifestyle: the (exclusively male) contingent was not allowed to marry during their tenure, lest their attention be diverted from the practice of medicine. Conditions for residents have become less draconian since those early days, though true-to-life narratives by young doctors continue to describe some rather harrowing initiation rites involved in becoming a doctor.[9] In 2010, the work-hours for residents are still very long, with thirty hours of continuous patient care duties every third night considered acceptable.[10]

The first year of residency training is termed **internship.** One of the primary purposes of internship is to expose the newly minted M.D. to as many patients as possible within their chosen field: to see every problem, to prescribe every course of treatment, and to perform every procedure. For this reason, **interns** are placed on the front lines of medical care. Although management of each patient is ultimately supervised by more senior doctors, interns perform the initial history and physical exam, write all of the orders, and get first crack at bedside procedures. Every July 1, a new batch of interns (who were medical students just a month ago) suddenly find themselves in the role of being someone's doctor. In the long course of medical education, the intern year is widely considered to be the most challenging.

As the **resident** progresses through second year and beyond, the level of comfort with patient care increases, and the resident begins to assume responsibility for managing more patients on her own. With more autonomy and graduated responsibility over the course of time, the junior resident becomes the senior resident, supervising medical students, interns and junior residents, effectively managing a team of patients.

During the entire training process, the resident still functions under the oversight and supervision of a fully trained physician, known in academic medical centers as the **attending.** The attending signs off on all momentous decisions (for example, major procedures, admission and discharge from the hospital), and bears ultimate responsibility for the patient's management. In academic hospitals, residents are the workhorses, so if you get seen in the ER there or are admitted to stay overnight, you will have a resident physician taking care of you, with the attending supervising the overall care.

Dr. Wen: I'm a senior resident now, at the fourth—and last—year of my training, and I can tell you that internship and residency are hard. It's not

---

✚ 911 ACTION TIP

When you go to a hospital and you are not sure who is talking to you, ask them directly, "Are you a student, resident, or attending?" A student or resident will say who they are, and often add their level of training (e.g., an intern versus senior resident). An attending will also not be shy to point out who they are (and may even be flattered that you think she could be young enough to be a student). You are entitled to know who is providing your medical care.

just that the hours are long—as brutal as it sounds, working twelve hours a day, six days a week, or not seeing your family and friends for thirty hours at a time, is something you get used to after a while. It's more the sheer amount of work that needs to be done under extreme time pressure. There's the expectation to keep on getting faster and faster while not letting any balls drop, and being able to see three, then seven, then a dozen sick patients all at once. I see it in myself, and I've seen it in my colleagues, that to save time, we do things like limiting the patient history to a short list of yes-or-no questions, going into each patient's room with a set framework in mind and kind of forcing the patient to fit into it.

A patient who comes in with vague symptoms, for example, is hard to deal with, because what does it mean that they are "just not feeling well"? It's tempting to stop listening and instead begin a fishing expedition. Shortness of breath? No. Abdominal pain? No. Chest pain? Well, once in a while. . . . Chest pain! Now that's something we know what to do with. Instead of taking the time to listen and actually figure out what's wrong, it's so much easier to latch on to a symptom and go with that. I'm not saying this is the right way to do things at all, but I do think that time pressure makes it seem easier to justify practicing, cookbook medicine.

Dr. Kosowsky: What Leana says is true; I saw it in myself as I went through residency, and I see it in my residents when all they can think about doing is getting their work done so they can finish and get some sleep. It's tempting to approach each patient as a checklist, to plug a series of yes-or-no answers into a formula and emerge with a plan.

Interestingly, I see a difference as the trainee moves from medical student to resident. The medical student is much more tolerant of open-ended questions and narrative-based interviews. The resident is harried and often just wants to "get on with it." But in asking only a prescribed set of questions, the resident misses important keys to diagnosis.[11]

It's part of our job as attending physicians to teach residents that there is a better way to approach patient care. The problem is that many attendings have been trained to take these shortcuts themselves, and have gotten so far from individualizing patient care that they don't see the problem. They reinforce the bad habits of cookbook medicine because the residents look up to

---

+ 911 ACTION TIP

*If you are not comfortable with the advice provided by a student or resi-
dent,* or if they are unable to answer your questions, you should ask to
speak to their attending.

---

attendings as their role models. So the human touch, the art of medicine,
and the fundamental importance of the diagnosis—these get lost during
the residency training process as it is today, and for many doctors, it is never
really regained.

At the end of residency, graduates become **attending** physicians. Some
may choose to further sub-specialize.[12] A **fellow** is someone who has completed residency and has embarked on additional, post-residency training
(for example, in cardiology or gastroenterology). Some fields, including
emergency medicine, do not require fellowships. The majority of residency
graduates do not pursue fellowships; they go directly to work as attendings.
Some decide to practice in the community and do not have teaching responsibilities. Others choose to work in academic hospitals, advancing research
and training the next generation of doctors.[13]

This is the general framework of medical education in the United States
today. This is how 16,000 medical students become resident doctors and
then attendings every year.[14] Physician and medical historian Dr. Kenneth
Ludmerer has referred to American medical education as one of the most
successful models of adult education in existence.[15] We agree. In many ways,
it is exemplary in how it has combined teaching with research and service
to society. The current U.S. system is the model of medical education that is
emulated throughout the world; indeed, every year, tens of thousands of
foreign medical school graduates attempt to take the U.S. licensing exams
in an effort to gain entrance to U.S. medical training.

Compare the existing state of affairs to how Abraham Flexner found
American medical education when he traveled across the country one hundred years ago. Medical schools had existed in the United States since the late
1700s, with the University of Pennsylvania, Harvard University, and Johns

Hopkins University among the first universities to have an affiliated medical school. Medical education became a lucrative business as more and more students sought to gain entrance. Unfortunately, there were few standards for what constituted a "medical school," and by the late 1800s, for-profit enterprises masquerading as educational institutions had proliferated by the dozens. This is an account of what Flexner saw when he audited some of these establishments:[16]

> *These enterprises—for the most part, they can be called schools or institutions only by courtesy—were frequently set up regardless of opportunity or need, in small towns as readily as in large, and at times, almost in the heart of the wilderness. No field, however limited, was ever effectually preempted. Wherever and whenever the roster of untitled practitioners rose above half a dozen, a medical school was likely at any moment to be precipitated. Nothing was really essential but professors . . .*
>
> *The teaching was, except for a little anatomy, wholly didactic. The schools were essentially private ventures, money-making in spirit and object. Income was simply divided among the lecturers, who reaped a rich harvest besides, through the consultations which the loyalty of their former students threw into their hands. . . . No applicant for instruction who could pay his fees or sign his note was turned down. . . . Accordingly, the business throve.*

Flexner also had some critical things to say about the few legitimate medical schools that he visited. About Harvard Medical School, he noted:[17]

> *The stethoscope had been in use for over thirty years before its first mention in the catalogue of the Harvard Medical School in 1868–69; the microscope is first mentioned the following year.*

At the end of the report, Flexner made three major recommendations, all three of which form the basis of how U.S. medical education functions today. First, he recommended that there be no more for-profit schools, and that all existing schools be linked to universities and teaching hospitals. Second, the students admitted must meet certain qualifications, including a rigorous undergraduate science education. Third, Flexner believed that scientific research should form the basis of all medical school teaching, and that medicine should be taught by those who are actively involved in original scientific investigation.[18]

Flexner's report was damning. Its recommendations spread like wildfire. Because the report addressed the lay public, there was public outrage about sham schools and quacks profiteering at the expense of the health and well-being of the nation. Not surprisingly, the impact was swift and significant: from 1910 to 1935, 89 of the 155 institutions that Flexner surveyed closed their doors. As the number of medical schools decreased, admission became more competitive and only students with qualified undergraduate degrees were granted entrance. The intertwining of medical training with universities and academic medical centers became complete. Medical students would receive training at university-affiliated teaching hospitals rather than at local clinics or home-based apprenticeship settings. Medical schools and their affiliated hospitals were to become engines of cutting-edge research, and medical training would be at the forefront of science.

In the first half of the twentieth century, this system of integrating teaching, clinical care, and scientific investigation worked well.[19] Clinical research was still predicated on direct interaction with patients, and those most gifted in clinical research tended to be the most talented clinicians and teachers. However, as scientific advances became increasingly specialized and technology-based, the cutting edge of science transitioned more and more from the wards to the laboratory. Those who were first-rate clinician-teachers found it difficult to also be first-rate researchers, and vice versa.[20]

As a result, the system in academic medical centers has become such that those who rise to the top tend to be the most productive researchers, not the ones most devoted to teaching clinical skills. Medical students and residents are no longer being taught diagnosis by expert physicians who have the talent or the passion for clinical teaching.[21] The apprentice model, where students learned at the feet of a master physician, has faded away.

The gradual erosion of teaching the art of medicine has contributed to the current Era of Depersonalized—and cookbook—Diagnosis. Understanding the scientific foundation for diagnostic principles is important, but by having scientists rather than clinicians define medical education, the art of diagnosis is becoming extinct. Clinical diagnosis is no longer an art passed down from master to apprentice, but rather as a recitation of recipes.

Dr. Wen: I attended one of the best medical schools in the country, Washington University School of Medicine. Our curriculum, which is quite typical of medical schools across the United States exemplifies what I call the post-Flexnerian ideal. Our first year was coursework focused on the normal workings of the human body: biochemistry, anatomy, physiology, and histology. In second year, we moved on to pathophysiology (or what happens when things go wrong) and system by system: the heart, the lungs, the gastrointestinal tract, etc. Every class was systemically structured. We went through thousands of diseases. For each disease, we learned how it was caused, how to diagnose it, how to treat it, how to prevent it. Every lecture was meticulously researched with professors presenting the latest theories and treatment advances. Typically, the lecturer would be a nationally renowned scientist doing cutting-edge research in that field.

Out of the dozens of courses in first and second year, we had just one class that addressed the human aspect of medicine. At Washington University, it was called the Practice of Medicine, or POM. All of us students loved POM. POM was where we learned how to interview patients and how to do the physical exam. We followed doctors to the bedside of patients and watched them do the interview, then we practiced it on each other and then on real patients. We learned how these expert doctors dealt with difficult situations like death, or medical error, or challenging patient and family dynamics. We read great physician-writers like William Carlos Williams and Oliver Sacks. More than ten years after I took the course, POM still stands out among the dozens of medical school courses because it was such a rare experience in my medical training. It's this art of medicine, and learning and seeing how medicine is practiced, that makes us doctors. That makes us human.

Dr. Kosowsky: I lead the equivalent of the POM course at Harvard Medical School.[22] My students really enjoy the course and they frequently comment that it's what makes the science and theory they learn seem relevant. After teaching thousands of students, I'm convinced that the majority of medical students enter their training with the right mind-set. They may be more inclined toward science than doctors of past generations, but in general, they understand that there is an art to medicine, and they want to be good diagnosticians and great doctors. The problem is that our medical education is often disproportionately focused on science and technology, and the desire to be an excellent clinician isn't nurtured or fostered.

If anything, it seems that the fundamentals of diagnostic reasoning are gradually eroded over the course of medical training. Here's a depressing anecdote. I teach first-year medical students in my course about the importance of the patient narrative. I ask students to take as much time as they want to listen to and appreciate the whole story; then we work together to see how a diagnosis emerges from the story. The students are impressed by the power of the narrative. They may not know all the medical terminology or arrive at the full diagnosis on their own, but they all "get" it: that the diagnosis naturally follows from the story.

Unfortunately, when these same students come to me as residents, they are less capable. They may know more about specific diagnoses, but they have lost the patience to listen to a patient's story. They'd rather use a recipe or go down a checklist of yes-or-no questions. Their range of diagnostic possibilities becomes more limited. They can't tolerate the uncertainty in the patient's story, so they take shortcuts and force the diagnostic process down narrow pathways—and in doing so, they often miss the key to the diagnosis.

This is a shame. We are failing the future generations of doctors. Medical training is supposed to make people into better doctors, not worse. But when budding doctors lose the ability to take a patient's history, diagnosis becomes dissociated from narrative, and it's no wonder the humanistic aspect gets lost in modern medicine. Doctors are no longer conditioned to listen, to think, to diagnose. Medical training, with its overemphasis on science to the exclusion of the art, is largely to blame.

Flexner himself recognized the problem with the overemphasis on science. Within fifteen years of issuing his report, Flexner wrote that medical education should also emphasize the interpersonal and humanistic aspects of care.[23]

Another reason for the decreasing emphasis on humanism in medicine is the decline of the apprenticeship method of learning. In the days of Sir William Osler and the Golden Era of Medical Diagnosis, medical training was an apprenticeship, with a student following a master clinician for up to a dozen years. The apprentice accompanied the master to patient care visits at the bedside; discussed each patient with the master; read the master's manuscripts; and submitted to the master's daily quizzing. To be sure, the education obtained at many of the for-profit schools that Flexner condemned was undoubtedly very poor. However, much was also lost in the new system of education where the institution of the medical school supplanted the master clinician as the primary pedagogue. Medical training has necessarily become more about science and technology, and recipes and algorithms, and less about the healing and the intangible things that can only be learned by observing a master in his daily practice.

Dr. Wen: Like other residents, I came to medical training to gain knowledge, learn skills, and perform life-saving procedures. I also came to residency to learn how expert doctors think. Medical training is not just about acquiring encyclopedic knowledge or mastering technical skills; it's also about learning the thought process behind medical decision-making, like how to conduct a patient interview, how to interpret signs and symptoms, and how to engage with patients of all ages and backgrounds.

Dr. Kosowsky: This is all part of the art of medicine that is so important, yet so little emphasized nowadays. It's human nature to want yes-or-no, clear-cut answers. I tell trainees that it can be uncomfortable to deal with the subtleties and uncertainties that accompany something so complex as human physiology (not to mention psychology!). This may be why listening to the patient's story can be so hard for doctors, because it introduces these shades of gray and the nuances that we aren't prepared to deal with, unless we've had a lot of practice. This is the kind of practice that medical training should do more to emphasize.

Arguably, the problems with modern medical training begin even before medical school. Reflecting Flexner's emphasis on academic excellence in the sciences, the medical school selection process tends to favor those who excel in math and science and perform well on tests, but not necessarily those who relate well to patients or are committed to service. Over time, this has led to a public health crisis. The United States is facing a serious undersupply of primary care physicians.[24] This shortage is acutely felt in rural and urban underserved areas. Recent reports have attributed these trends to the lack of service inclination among medical school matriculants and the inadequacy of fostering the sense of duty to society during medical school and residency.[26]

In recent years, some educators have come to recognize the importance of learning the art of diagnosis, and there are renewed efforts to provide one-on-one mentorship in both medical school and residency. In some training programs, there is the option to train in community-health sites, and medical students are even encouraged to do home visits with expert clinicians, just like in the old days.[25]

There are renewed calls to reform the way that medical students are recruited and trained so that those in the medical profession are not just smart and knowledgeable of the sciences, but also dedicated to service and society.[27] This, in fact, is what Flexner would have wanted. A section of the seminal report that is almost always overlooked is his writing on the physician's social contract: commitment to service, professionalism, and the individual patient. A hundred years after his report, we feel confident in saying that Abraham Flexner would have been proud of his overall impact on medical education—but disheartened at several of his report's unintended consequences.

To celebrate the one-hundred-year anniversary of the Flexner report, a group of twenty-five young health professionals around the world came together to propose a new set of reforms in medical education.[28] These changes are long overdue. They begin with selection of future doctors who are committed to service and the patient-doctor relationship, future doctors who are open to a role not just as scientists but as healers. They continue through medical school where the ideals of physicians' commitment to patients and society should be fostered and nurtured. Residency presents further opportunities for targeted learning to take place, such as the reemergence of apprenticeship models of learning.

The Flexner-era changes to American medical training moved medicine forward in many ways, but also helped to derail the art of diagnosis and usher in a modern era of algorithmic thinking and depersonalized care. Now, in a time of rapid reform, there is a real opportunity to not just improve access to healthcare, but also to make significant improvements to how future doctors are trained and to reaffirm what medicine is supposed to be about: to serve patients and society.

911 REVIEW

- Medical training involves multiple transitions: from premedical student to medical student, to intern, resident, and then attending physician.
- Abraham Flexner introduced many reforms to revolutionize U.S. medical education, but there were also several unintended consequences that propagated cookbook medicine.
- One hundred years after Flexner, as medical education is once again undergoing reform, we have a real opportunity to refocus medical training to care for patients and society.

Part II

Cookbook Medicine—
Live from the ER

Cookbook medicine has an intrinsically negative ring to it. If a doctor were to advertise that she practiced using a cookbook approach to diagnosis, following a fixed recipe for each patient, it's doubtful that patients would come flocking. No one would argue that doctors should be knowledgeable about best practices and keep up-to-date on the latest guidelines. There may even be a role for algorithms when it comes to treating straightforward conditions such as colds and sore throats.[1] But ultimately, we want to be treated like individuals. This is common sense.

If it's so obvious that cookbook medicine is bad, why is it so tolerated? Why do patients put up with it? And what can they do to get their doctors to change?

To begin to answer these questions, we take you through four real-life examples of cookbook medicine. Our cases come live from the ER, but they could have happened in your child's pediatrician's office or the inpatient ward where your parent is hospitalized. Through the cases, we demonstrate the thought process of the cookbook physician and the impact of cookbook medicine on patients, doctors, and the healthcare system. We describe each case from the point of view of the patient, the doctor, the nurse, and other healthcare providers, as we highlight the pitfalls of cookbook thinking. Our ✚ *911 Action Tips direct you to be on the lookout for these pitfalls.*

As you read through the chapters, put yourself in the shoes of the healthcare providers and consider what it is that makes them default to practicing cookbook medicine. Then think about yourself in the shoes of the patient. What diagnostic approach would you have wanted? How could you have better directed the situation to get the care that you deserve?

Three

The Car Mechanic with the Pulled Muscle

We are already well acquainted with our mechanic, Jerry, the out-of-shape forty-eight-year-old who was moving boxes and got worried about his chest tightness. Let's begin our discussion with him.

First, a quick introduction to the other professionals that Jerry encountered that day. Before you see a doctor, you typically have to navigate through a series of other individuals who work in the hospital. In the ER, like most other outpatient settings, this usually begins with a **receptionist,** who checks you in and takes basic information such as your date of birth, home address, and insurance information. The next person you see may be a **patient care tech.** These techs are referred to by a number of other terms, including medical assistant, nurse's aid, clinical care associate, or clinical assistant. Techs receive training to assist with basic duties, such as obtaining vital signs (heart rate, blood pressure, temperature, and so on), and setting up for bedside tests such as EKGs and pelvic exams. They also can help patients with disrobing, toileting, and other necessities.

At some point early on, you'll probably see a **nurse.** Nurses are licensed professionals who have at least two years of healthcare training. In the ER, there is often one nurse appointed to be the **triage nurse,** seeing all the patients as they come in and deciding who needs to be seen next. The triage nurse will conduct an initial assessment by asking you questions and

---

✚ 911 ACTION TIP

If you are unsure of who is asking you questions, interrupt her and ask her who she is. A short and direct question, "And you are . . . ?" will do the trick.

---

performing a brief physical exam. Depending on the practice setting, they may draw blood or order certain tests, such as an EKG. Eventually, you'll see a **doctor,** who will form his or her own assessment and order additional testing or treatment. It's then up to the team—nurses, techs, and others—to help carry out the plan.[1]

Now that we know who these individuals are, let's see what is going through their minds, and Jerry's, as he arrives in the ER.

Triage nurse: My job is to see all patients when they first come to the ER; that way, if someone looks really sick, I can make sure the doctor sees them sooner. One of the things we're trained to do is document why someone is there and boil it down to one or two words, which we call the "**chief complaint.**"

In Jerry's case, it's easy. His chief complaint, the reason he came to the ER, is chest pain. I'll go on to ask some more questions, but when I hear chest pain, I'm thinking, this could be life-threatening, because chest pain might be a heart attack. So that immediately activates our "chest pain protocol." Even though Jerry didn't look that "sick," I know that looks can fool you. That means Jerry doesn't just sit there in the waiting room along with the sore throat or the sprained ankle: he comes back immediately with a tech and we get the tests going.

Jerry: Before I know what's going on, they're undressing me and putting stickers on my chest. I get worried, you know, because I didn't think this was that serious. Was it something I said to the nurse? I thought I mentioned that the pain felt more like a muscle spasm and actually was getting better. But then all of a sudden everyone's in a big hurry, as if every minute counted. I'm thinking: I'm glad I didn't wait any longer at home! Nobody tells me what tests they're going to do, but I trust them. I figured I'd be there for a couple of hours to wait for the doctor to see me and get the test results back.

Patient care tech: From the moment the triage nurse told me about this guy, I knew he was going to be there all night. Whenever some middle-aged man comes in with anything like chest pain, the "chest pain pathway" gets activated. This includes the EKG that I do as soon as they come in, a chest X-ray, and the lab tests looking for heart damage: the cardiac enzymes. Once one set of enzymes is checked, the "pathway" is that we have to draw blood in several hours to check the enzymes again. This also means that these patients stay for a stress test in the morning to make sure there's no problem. It's all part of the "chest pain pathway," so nobody questions that that's what this guy is getting.

Jerry: After the initial flurry of activity, it seems like things are back to business as usual. Lots of waiting. Lots of people coming in and asking the same questions over and over. By this time, no one seems overly concerned that I'm having a heart attack. At one point the doctor tells me everything looked fine. But the way he makes it sound, there's no way to be sure unless I stay all night. I really want to leave, but they keep on saying it's not safe, and I don't want to argue. I mean, what if I go home and have a heart attack? So I decide to stay. I'm worried about those hospital bills though. I don't think my wife and I have the greatest insurance coverage, and I know this is going to cost our family.

Doctor: Every day, I see two, three, sometimes more patients like Jerry. We do more or less the same thing. Does the "chest pain pathway" get activated more than it should? Probably. Actually, we know that very few, if any, of these patients will ultimately turn out to have heart attacks. But as doctors, we always have to think about the worst-case scenario. A middle-aged, overweight man with chest pain? That's a heart attack until proven otherwise. We need algorithms and pathways in place to catch one-in-a-thousand cases, or else that's a big lawsuit coming my way if I miss it. I don't have time to sort through and find the needle in the haystack, even if that were possible, which I'm not sure it is. So, at the end of the day, I order a few extra tests, nobody will fault me, or my hospital, for playing it safe. That's why these "chest pain pathways" work for me.

After hearing this story from everyone's point of view, it's still hard not to feel empathy toward Jerry. You might feel indignant toward the providers, and toward a system, where blind obedience to pathways is acknowledged openly. When multiplied by hundreds of thousands of patients, it's not hard to see how this results in a healthcare system with out-of-control costs.

So what went wrong and how can we change it? Let's start by working through this case. We will identify some specific pitfalls of cookbook medicine and show you how to address them head on.

In Jerry's case, it all began with the *misplaced emphasis on the chief complaint*.[2] The premise of a chief complaint is that a patient's story can be boiled down to one or two words, a single phrase selected from among a list of common symptoms: chest pain, headache, weakness, shortness of breath, etc. This is a familiar strategy in many aspects of our lives. When we dial the toll-free service line for the cable company, we hear the familiar prompts: for billing questions, press "1"; for changes to your service, press "2"; and so forth. The same thing happens at the nurse's station: for chest pain, go here; for abdominal pain, go there.

There's an appealing simplicity to this strategy. But that's exactly the problem. It's not just that stock phrases don't capture the complexity of a patient's story (after all, there is plenty of opportunity in the medical record to delve into further detail); it's that the chief complaint becomes a proxy for the patient's story, setting in motion a course of action that may or may not have any real relevance for the individual patient. "Chest pain" signals something to the tech, the other nurses, and the doctor that is very different than the story itself. It doesn't require medical training to appreciate that Jerry's description of chest tightness after moving boxes might mean something different than another patient's description of chest pain! Yet the initial designation of Jerry as having "chest pain" triggers a set of responses on the part of all of the providers that became difficult to redirect.

In Chapter 8, we discuss the chief complaint in much more detail and show how patients can get their doctors to think beyond it. Moving on, we

---

✚ 911 ACTION TIP

Beware when a particular response raises alarm in your nurse or doctor. Ask them what it is and why. This is a good opportunity to clarify before they put all their emphasis on this "chief complaint." (It may also be a good lesson for you to know what your doctor considers a worrisome symptom or finding.)

---

identify the second pitfall in Jerry's case to be *the path always traveled*. Virtually every ER has diagnostic pathways or protocols for major complaints. To save time, there may be standardized "order sets" implemented such that as soon as a patient comes in with a certain complaint, a defined set of lab tests or imaging tests are ordered. Abdominal pain? There are standard labs to go with that, plus or minus an ultrasound or a CT scan. Chest pain? There is the standard chest X-ray, EKG, and blood work. Headache? There are set labs and imaging studies. Chief complaints get protocolized into a pathway, a recipe for a set list of things that must follow.

There is a reason why ERs traditionally rely so heavily on pathways. It wasn't long ago that the ER was truly the backwater of medicine. If you were unfortunate enough to present to an ER with a serious problem a generation ago, you probably would have seen an intern learning on the job with little to no supervision. Often, it was the triage nurse who had the most experience; it was up to her to decide who was sick and who wasn't, who could wait to be seen by their private physician and who needed a specialist called in. Because there weren't enough trained doctors to look after patients in ERs, it was up to the triage nurse who had to get things going without a doctor's orders —hence the emergence of pathways to make sure something was being done to help these ER patients.[3]

Thankfully, times have changed. Now, emergency medicine is a full-fledged specialty with physicians who are residency trained and board certified in acute care and medical and trauma resuscitation. However, pathways are still commonplace in the ER and other practice settings. In Jerry's case, there was no good reason to preemptively initiate any kind of pathway. If a thoughtful doctor had heard his story when he first came in, he wouldn't have needed any tests at all. Yet, once the triage nurse flagged him as having "chest pain," it was off to the races. There were labs and an X-ray. Then, because one set of blood work was drawn, and Jerry was already flagged as being part of the "chest pain pathway," it became more difficult to stop the pathway from progressing. Inertia is a powerful force, and medicine is no exception; to keep going is easy, but stopping midway through the pathway requires more justification. This becomes a depersonalized and wasteful way to practice medicine.

Dr. Wen: My colleagues around the country tell me that many of their ERs, hospitals, and clinics have these pathways. When a patient comes in with a "chief complaint" that matches a pathway, it gets activated—often before seeing a doctor. The thought behind a system like this is that it saves time and improves efficiency; the labs and tests are back by the time the doctor sees the patient, so faster decisions can be made.

Perhaps this system is more efficient for doctors (even this contention is one that I don't agree with, but more on this later). But it better for patients? Well, sometimes, efficiency can help. Let's say a woman comes in complaining of burning when she urinates: a urine test can be sent right away to determine if she has a urinary tract infection. That makes sense—when she sees the doctor, the doctor already knows the result of the test and can prescribe antibiotics, if necessary. That's more efficient overall.

However, most cases are more complex than this. What if the chief complaint is dizziness or abdominal pain—something that doesn't lend itself easily to one test? Or, consider what happens when an abnormal result comes back on a test that wasn't really needed. Now, a test that may have no bearing on why the patient came in in the first place needs to be followed up with even more tests. Let's say that Jerry's blood tests were all normal, except for a slightly elevated white blood cell count. Typically, doctors think of white blood cells being increased in the presence of an infection. Does this mean Jerry has an infection that needs to be accounted for? Not necessarily, because elevated white blood cell count is extremely nonspecific, and can be found in any number of settings, including pain or stress. But once an abnormal result is found, the doctor may feel compelled to search for an infection, even though nothing else about Jerry's story suggested he had an infection. Whatever time the doctor "saved" on not listening to the story ends up being a lot more time for the patient to wait for additional tests.

Dr. Kosowsky: What happens, too, is that once you set off down a particular pathway, it becomes even harder to go back and think about what the patient actually has. Take the young woman who has burning with urination. The urinalysis comes back normal, so the patient is sent home reassured that "everything looks fine." But the real diagnosis—in this case let's say it's a sexually transmitted disease like chlamydia—is never made because she got started off on the wrong pathway.

Just last week, I saw a young woman who had been to two doctors for her belly pain and was told, after blood work and an ultrasound and two CTs, that they couldn't find anything wrong with her. But she continued to have abdominal pain, and it turned out to be from a stomach ulcer—something the doctors didn't have a pathway for. Pathways may help to **"rule out"** certain conditions, but they inevitably miss things. I'm uncomfortable with the whole notion of "ruling out" this or that diagnosis, as if that's the goal. Better to make the correct diagnosis, no?

The other phrase that drives me crazy is the **"workup."** Patients often hear that they are being "worked up" for a disease. You're getting the "workup" for heart attack or appendicitis. Again, this implies a single-minded focus on one pathway, one disease. That's not good medicine.

This brings us to the third pitfall in Jerry's case: the pitfall of *worst-case reasoning.* Thinking about the worst-case possibility is not inherently bad. It's something intuitive for ER doctors and boy scouts alike, because the whole idea is that they will be prepared if something bad does happen. It can also be easier for the doctor, because diagnosis goes from trying to figure

---

✚ 911 ACTION TIP

Beware of the diagnostic pathway. Look out when a doctor, a nurse, or a tech tells you that you are getting a test because it's a part of a "pathway." Ask your doctor to explain to you why you are getting a test and what he thinks it will help show.

out a differential diagnosis—that is, a list of possible diseases that could possibly account for the patient's symptoms—to simply excluding the one or two diagnoses that are the most life-threatening.

The problem arises when worst-case reasoning becomes the *only* reasoning. In Jerry's case, the "worst case" for a middle-aged man with chest pain immediately led all the care providers involved to think about a heart attack. Was it theoretically possible that Jerry was having a heart attack? Well, anything is *possible*. But his story really doesn't suggest it, and taking the time to hear it would have been enough to seal the deal. Not to mention, we can't always even predict what the worst-case scenario might be. In this sense, "worst-case scenario" reasoning forces doctors into pathways that can, paradoxically, keep them from making other important diagnoses that can be equally serious if missed.

The better question to ask is: was this scary diagnosis suggested by any part of Jerry's presentation? Given Jerry's story and physical exam, the single answer was "no." Doing further tests to make absolutely sure wasn't necessary; "playing it safe" is not justification alone. In everyday life, this approach would be equivalent to never getting in a car or airplane just because the worst-case scenario is a fatal crash. We don't live our lives based solely on fear, and we shouldn't tolerate medicine practiced that way, either.

Dr. Kosowsky: At some level, making a diagnosis comes down to common sense. One question I always like to ask residents and medical students is whether the diagnosis they are considering makes sense. Would it make sense that Jerry had pulled muscle? Well, he just moved a lot of heavy furniture; he feels like he has a pulled muscle; his pain was localized to a specific muscle group, and was worse when he tensed his muscles—sure, that would make sense. What about a heart attack? Again, anything is possible, but it

---

✚ 911 ACTION TIP

Beware when your doctor tells you that he has to "rule out" or "work up" a scary-sounding disease. Ask her what it is that she thinks you have, not just the worst-case scenario.

would be some coincidence that his presentation would almost exactly mimic a muscle strain right after moving his brother into his new apartment. So common sense tells you it's just not believable.

We will explain more about the concept of the differential diagnosis in Chapter 7, but you can see in this simple example that there are other modes of thinking beyond following a pathway based on a chief complaint and pursuing worst-case reasoning.

As we know, Jerry did not have a heart attack—though he did end up staying overnight in the hospital to get a stress test that was indeterminate. The only thing he learned in the end was that he was out of shape and couldn't finish the treadmill test—a fact that he didn't need much reminding. However, after going through all that and being told that the doctors still had no explanation for his pain, Jerry was worried and far from reassured. There was the hospital bill, for starters. As for his wife, who sent him in: she was angry. How could it be that her husband went to get all these tests and there was still no answer? If that's the case, it must be something serious.

Doctor: I'm not really surprised by the outcome. The chances of someone like Jerry having a heart attack are actually pretty miniscule. Even knowing the outcome, though, I'd do the same thing again. Following a recipe is easy and saves me time. It's the safe thing to do and protects me against malpractice. Also, we bill for the time patients spend overnight and the hospital is reimbursed for all the tests. So it's a no-brainer.

Jerry: What I don't get is why nobody discussed this whole decision process with me. I definitely wouldn't have stayed the night if my doctor had told me that he really didn't think I was having a heart attack, or that the additional tests were unlikely to show anything. I don't expect doctors to be perfect, but I do expect someone to give a bit of thought before shuttling me down some pathway.

Doctors can't be perfect. This doesn't, though, translate into a need for defensive, unnecessary tests just to prevent lawsuits. Quite the contrary. In order to establish malpractice, one has to prove that the doctor deviated from the standard of care.[4] The standard of care is defined by what other reasonably qualified doctors would have done in the same or similar circumstances. It's a common sense definition, that, while testified to by experts, is ultimately decided by a jury of laypeople. If a patient is showing obvious signs of heart attack and an electrocardiogram is never performed, that's a departure from the standard of care. But if the patient has a broken rib or a painful rash on his chest, there is no standard of care requiring that the doctor order every test in the book to exclude the possibility of a heart attack.

Dr. Wen: Our chairman at Brigham and Women's Hospital, Dr. Ron Walls, likes to say that the answer to preventing lawsuits isn't getting more tests: it's spending time with the patient to become more confident of your diagnosis. A number of studies have investigated this subject, and each time, they have found that overordering of tests doesn't lead to fewer malpractice claims, but rather, that more time with patients and better communication with them will. Shocking, right? More time and better communication leads to a more accurate diagnosis and better care, and ultimately, that should be our goal—not fewer lawsuits.

There's so much wrong with following cookie-cutter recipes that we haven't even touched upon yet. For example, let's say Jerry, in this case, was a smoker. He might also have had high cholesterol, and maybe was on the way to developing diabetes. If he were just sent home and told his heart was fine, he might still have a heart attack in a year or two because of his lifestyle habits. Telling a patient he didn't have a heart attack is false reassurance unless the doctor actually takes time to explain what symptoms mean and what else to watch out for.

Let's consider the reasons that proponents of cookbook medicine use for justifying their practice: it's easier, it's safer, and supposedly it saves time. The first reason may, in fact, be true; it probably is easier for the practitioner, but that's hardly a satisfying rationale. It may seem to be "safer" to try to rule out "life-threatening diseases," but as we will discuss in later chapters, tests are not perfect and can never provide 100 percent reassurance. One can also argue that excessive exposure to tests and radiation is not safer, and that ordering the test and blindly going down a pathway may miss the boat

---

✚ 911 ACTION TIP

Your doctor has multiple pressures to practice cookbook medicine. Try to change the conversation so it focuses on your diagnosis and what's best for you. Ask, "What is it that I have? How can you be sure? Why do you think so?"

---

altogether and an even more serious diagnosis might be overlooked. Finally, in terms of efficiency, we argue that in the long run, you'll save more time by getting to the right diagnosis, not by following blind alleyways that don't lead anywhere.

If you have flown on an airplane since 9/11, you can appreciate that cookbook medicine is not dissimilar to what occurs at airports around the country. The Transportation Security Administration instructs security screeners to follow the same routine so that everyone who walks to their plane gets asked the same questions ("Did you pack your bag yourself?") and goes through the same X-ray machines, regardless of whether the passenger is a little old lady with a walker or a young man wearing an Osama bin Laden shirt. All of us who have been to an airport recently can recite the recipe: laptops must be removed from your carry-on; all liquids and gels must be less than three ounces and in separate containers; jackets, belts, shoes have to come off; everything out of your pockets. Does treating everyone the same way really result in better outcomes? Common sense tells us "no." Studies have been shown that a tailored approach to screening such as that employed by Israel's El Al airlines is far more effective in achieving its aim of picking out the real "worst-case scenarios."[5]

The need for an individualized approach to diagnosis is the reason why no matter how sophisticated computers have become, they have not been able to replace doctors. IBM designed an artificial intelligence machine, named "Watson" that seemingly "understood" natural-language questions and was able to beat *Jeopardy* champions at their own game. Since then, Watson has been programmed to filter through a patient's various symptoms to try to come up with a diagnosis. But though Watson passes the test when given an abstract list of symptoms, it fails in actual patient encounters.

Many observers were shocked, but Dr. Atul Gawande, the author of *The Checklist Manifesto*, was not surprised.

"I think part of the bafflement occurs because the folks who know how to make such systems don't understand how the clinical encounter actually operates," said Dr. Gawande in an interview. He went on to discuss how the clinical encounter—and the individual patient—is far more complex than an algorithm can handle.[6] The founder of Watson himself, Dr. Herbert Chase, has acknowledged that there are complexities of the human condition that will always favor the astute doctor. "The computer is never going to be able to read the signals that the patient is emoting, like 'I don't really want to do that' or 'I'm a little afraid of that,'" Chase has said.[7]

Indeed, individual complexity has a lot to do with patient preferences around diagnostic certainty. A recent study found that patients have a wide range of tolerance when it comes to acceptable personal risk. Most people were willing to accept at least a 5 percent risk of an adverse outcome in order to forgo admission to the hospital, but some wanted to be admitted even if the risk was less than 0.5 percent. The researchers looked to see if they could find a pattern to predict which patients were more likely to be risk-tolerant or risk-adverse, but couldn't find any.[8]

So if doctors can't rely on premade pathways, if computer algorithms won't be providing us with the answers anytime soon, and if patients all have difference preferences, how can medical decisions be made? Here's a shocking answer. Listen to the patient and have an open and honest discussion! Interestingly, a study of patients with chest pain in the ER found that patients were far more likely to choose to go home than providers were to send them home. Whereas only 3 percent of physicians would send a patient home if there was a 5 percent or smaller chance of missing a heart attack, 43 percent of their patients who understood the risks would have opted to go home.[9] Such variation in preferences among patients should make it even more incumbent on doctors and patients to have a frank discussion and to make a decision together rather than adopting the cookbook route that treats all patients alike. Cookbook recipes may seem simpler for the doctor, but the patient will end up like Jerry, with more uncertainty and more anxiety.

So how do you avoid Jerry's fate? Read on. In the meantime, Jerry has some advice.

"Always ask your doctor what pathway they are using," he says. "Then ask that you get your own pathway and not just the recipe that every other patient follows."

911 REVIEW

- The pitfalls of cookbook medicine begin with the misplaced emphasis on the chief complaint, over-reliance on pathways and too much worst-case reasoning.
- Doctors have multiple pressures to practice cookbook medicine.
- To get the care you deserve, you need to challenge your doctor and make sure things are done based on your individual case and not based on a generic recipe.

Four

The Mother of Two Who Had Trouble Breathing

Meet Annette Golding. She is a thirty-two-year-old woman who lives in Marblehead, an upper-middle-class community north of Boston. Annette is the mother of eight-month-old Emma and three-year-old Todd. For as long as she could remember, Annette has had trouble controlling her weight. She was on the heavy side when she graduated from high school, and, in spite of her petite frame, her dress size has steadily gone up, no thanks to half-a-dozen fad diets.

"I know it's my fault, but it's hard, you know? I work at the desk all day, then I come home and cook dinner for my family. When I got pregnant for the second time, forget it, the weight kept climbing and I just gave up trying to keep it down." Her weight was up almost twenty pounds over the past year, and she was closing in on 250.

Aside from her weight problems and some mild asthma, Annette had been pretty healthy. A few months ago, she began finding it hard to stay awake during the day, to the point that she'd find herself taking cat-naps at red lights along her thirty-minute commute into Boston.

At night, she was a restless sleeper, although, until recently, that had a lot to do with the nightly disruptions to tend to breastfeeding and diaper changes. Now that her baby was sleeping through the night, she still didn't feel as if she was ever getting enough sleep. At the same time, she couldn't say she was suffering from insomnia; in fact, after a full day at work and chasing after the little ones, she was downright pooped by the time the kids were tucked in, and she would be asleep practically before her head hit the pillow.

Annette was also noticing that she was getting more out of breath climbing the two flights of stairs up to the kids' playroom, something she attributed to her weight gain and just being out of shape. She tried using her asthma inhaler a few times, but it didn't seem to help. After putting it off for weeks, she finally went to her doctor. She was hoping he might be able to prescribe some sort of energy pill, but he seemed much more focused on her asthma. He wrote her a prescription for a new inhaler, which she never got around to filling at the pharmacy.

Last week, Annette decided to travel up to Toronto to spend a weekend with her sister, who just recently had a new baby of her own.

"It was a good weekend," she recounts, "except I was so tired. I felt so self-conscious, too. They have a small apartment, and my sister and brother-in-law kept on making fun of me because my snoring woke them up from two rooms down." She hadn't known that she snored so loudly; her husband never mentioned it.

When she got back to Marblehead, she felt more tired than ever. One day, she nearly fell asleep driving with her kids from daycare. She knew that something had to be done. Her doctor was out of town, but she managed to get an appointment to see one of the other doctors in the office that day. She arrived at the office, anxious and out of breath, having chugged a double espresso in traffic and walked the last block to the medical building at a brisk pace. The new doctor held her chart in his hand and inquired about her shortness of breath—which by her account was no better. He asked her about the last time she was hospitalized for asthma (not since she was a teenager), about any recent travel (nothing other than for the trip to Toronto), about her history of smoking (she had smoked cigarettes briefly while in college), about chest pain and palpitations she didn't have either. He inquired more about her asthma. She didn't want to admit that the prescription for the new inhaler was still folded up in her pocketbook.

The new doctor took a stethoscope to her lungs and asked her to breathe deeply in out through her mouth before announcing his verdict: "No wheezing; your lungs are clear." Initially she thought this would be good news. How bad could her asthma be if this doctor couldn't even hear any wheezing? But it wasn't good news. The doctor told her that he was actually very worried, and wanted an ambulance to take her to the ER to get a CT scan of her lungs.

"Obese smoker, birth control pills, recent plane trip, persistent SOB—rule out PE," he wrote on the referral sheet. Meaning that because she had "risk factors" and persistent shortness of breath, he wanted to "rule out" pulmonary embolism (PE), or a blood clot in the lungs.

Annette: What just happened was a blur. I didn't get what my doctor was saying. OK, I have to lose weight. I get it. But smoking? Was that on my chart? I mean, when I was in college, I smoked some cigarettes at parties, but that hardly makes me a smoker. And birth control? I used to take the Pill, but then after I got married, I stopped. Otherwise how do I have two young kids!

Up until now, I haven't been all that worried about my breathing. It's this tiredness that brought me in. But the doctor seemed to just focus on my breathing, which isn't that bad. He didn't really explain why I needed to go to the ER, other than saying there was something that could be very dangerous. Then the ambulance came. I got really scared. Wouldn't you have?

Triage nurse: I wrote down exactly what the referral slip said. It was this woman's own doctor's office who referred her. Nurses are supposed to do assessments and describe what's going on, but this sounded to me like a textbook case of PE. When the ambulance brings this woman to triage, she's breathing OK and she's talking a mile a minute, so deep down I'm not too worried. What I found strange is how she goes on about being tired. That's such a minor issue compared to a PE.

Doctor: Before I see this patient, I read the nurse's note and the referring doctor's note. I mean, this woman has a pretty good story for a PE. She's short of breath; she has a lot of the risk factors. That's what's written on the chart. Her heart rate is just on the borderline of being high, and her oxygen saturation on room air is on the low side of normal. That's all consistent with a blood clot. PE is a life-threatening condition, and it's the very first thing I think of. I tell Annette we need to do a CT scan of her lungs right away to see if she had a blood clot. But she refuses.

Annette: No, I don't want a CT scan![1] I've read a lot about CT scans. I know about the risks they can cause in terms of radiation exposure. My mother had Hodgkin's lymphoma, which they thought was from radiation treatments to her thyroid when she was young. So I ask the ER doctor if there are any other options.

Doctor: We make a compromise. We can start with some blood work and a chest X-ray. There's a test called the d-dimer test, which is a screening test we can do. It's just a blood test. If it's negative, it's reassuring. If it's positive, then we have to be more worried.

Annette: I appreciate that this doctor is willing to listen to my opinion. I'm not sure he really wanted to listen to my story, though. I try to explain that I wasn't really that short of breath but mostly just tired. I tell him maybe I'm tired because my sister was making me self-conscious about my snoring, but he doesn't think this is funny, or maybe he doesn't hear it. He's not interested. It's as if he made up his mind already that all he has to do is make sure I don't have a PE.

Doctor: As it turns out, I was right to be worried. The d-dimer blood test is positive. That means we have to do a CT scan to rule out PE.

Nurse: I knew from the moment this woman came in that she'd be getting a CT scan. Her risk factors are so obvious. Anyway, so she gets the CT after all. It's unfortunate, really. The scan isn't great quality because of her size. There isn't an obvious PE, but the radiologists say that they can't be 100 percent sure.

Annette: I don't remember the rest of that day; maybe I just blocked it all out as some really bad memory. I do remember the doctor saying that the CT scan is incomplete, and they can't be sure that there's no blood clot. They did find something else on the CT, though someone mentioned the "C" word—cancer. That got me pretty scared.

Doctor: On the CT, we see what looks like a nodule in her lung, which could mean anything. In someone who is young and otherwise healthy, it's probably not cancer. But she was a smoker, so it's important for her to go through more tests and make sure it's benign. It's something that definitely needs follow-up. In the meantime, she still has to be admitted to the hospital because we still can't be sure it's not a PE.

Annette: So it's not bad enough that I get one CAT scan. They tell me that I have to stay in the hospital, get more studies, and see more doctors. So I do. I stay in the hospital for five whole days. They do all kinds of tests, including another CT of my lungs and an ultrasound of my heart and another one of my legs. I keep hearing that the tests were hard to interpret because of my "body habitus," which I guess is a nicer-sounding way for saying I'm too fat for them to get the right results. I get so many vials of blood taken that I felt weak. They call in a general internist and a specialist in infectious diseases and then a heart specialist and a nutritionist. Nobody can figure out what's wrong with me.

I finally get discharged, and for several weeks, I get referrals to see even more doctors. I have a lung biopsy where they go in and take a piece of the nodule they saw on CT. All this time, I'm feeling exhausted, but I don't know if it's just because I'm so tired of all those tests and scared because I don't know what was going on. When they mention that perhaps I should see a psychiatrist, I begin to think maybe it really is all in my head!

Annette's ordeal came to an end when one of her doctors took a particular interest in her trip to Toronto—not the airplane trip itself, but in what her sister had said about her snoring. He recognized that her constellation of symptoms pointed to a diagnosis of obstructive sleep apnea (OSA). OSA is due to the collapse of the upper airway during sleep—something we experience as snoring. In extreme cases, this results in periods of apnea, in which breathing stops entirely and oxygen in the bloodstream drops precipitously. Patients with OSA can have hundreds of episodes where they stop breathing every night, causing restless sleep and daytime exhaustion.

OSA is a common problem, affecting up to 4 percent of women and 9 percent of men.[2] It is particularly common in individuals who are overweight or obese. Making the diagnosis of OSA is important, because it is a reversible disease that can be treated, and because, unless it's reversed, it can have serious long-term negative consequences including permanent damage to the lungs and progressive heart failure. It can also have significant negative effects on lifestyle and, as Annette was afraid of, the danger of increased fatigue in causing motor vehicle accidents.

There are three major signs of OSA: snoring, excessive daytime sleepiness, and report by significant others of sleep apnea episodes. Annette was not aware of her snoring until her sister mentioned it, but she certainly had the excessive sleepiness—that was her main problem and the reason she sought medical care in the first place. As for the report by others, her doctors hadn't asked for her husband's side of things. When they did, he said, in fact, that her breathing was "strange" at night and she often appeared to stop breathing altogether. She always did breathe eventually, though, so he hadn't thought that much about it. And her snoring?

"Of course I knew! I'm not deaf," he said. "I just couldn't bring it up. She doesn't know this, but I've been sleeping with earplugs every night."

In looking back, all of the symptoms needed to diagnose OSA were there from the very first visit she made to her primary care physician. Annette's obesity, her daytime drowsiness, and her shortness of breath certainly fit the pattern for OSA. However, several factors conspired to push the diagnosis of pulmonary embolism—the worst-case scenario—to the forefront. As a result, all kinds of tests got ordered, in the ER and thereafter. Annette had far more radiation exposure than she had wanted, or needed. She had months of nail-biting angst when her problems could have been resolved from the first visit. She had a significant delay in diagnosis of a serious problem—a disease that afflicts at least one in twenty people, as compared to the much rarer pulmonary embolism at one in a thousand people. So why wasn't the diagnosis made earlier by the many doctors who saw her?

Let's start with what happened that day in the ER. Because of what the primary care doctor wrote on the referral slip, the triage nurse and then the doctor focused on the need to "r/o PE"—to "rule out" this worst-case of a pulmonary embolism. Even after Annette explained that she did not have the risk factors that they thought she had in terms of smoking, birth control pills, and travel, they still considered her to be high risk.[3] The entire slew of tests she had in the ER was aimed at making sure she *didn't* have one particular disease.

This pitfall of *diagnostic momentum* is a significant danger in cookbook medicine. When one doctor identifies a potential diagnosis, other doctors tend to focus on that diagnosis to the exclusion of others. It is much easier to go with the history that was already taken than to start from scratch. Yet, the initial history was incomplete and led the primary care doctor, then the ER team and a whole host of specialists, down the wrong path.

The problems of diagnostic momentum started with the primary care doctor. Perhaps he was in a hurry. Perhaps he focused exclusively on one system for some reason. Whatever happened in the initial office visit, the diagnostic approach was one that overemphasized part of the history (the shortness of breath) while leaving out other important components (the fatigue, the

---

✚ 911 ACTION TIP

Beware when your doctor seems to be relying on someone else's impressions. Ask your doctor, "What do *you* think is going on?" If she says the same thing as your previous doctor, ask her if you can tell your story from the beginning. Tell her that you came to her because you trust her judgment and you want her to hear the whole story from you herself. This encourages the second doctor to start from scratch and formulate her own opinions.

snoring, the gradual onset of symptoms that started *before* the travel). The subsequent momentum led the ER doctor to rely on the primary care doctor; the specialists on the floor to rely on the ER doctor; and so on. While it may seem efficient to see another doctor's thought process, relying on it exclusively leads to premature, incomplete, and often incorrect diagnoses.

Dr. Kosowsky: Part of what I think went wrong with Annette's case is the failure of pattern recognition. Expert doctors are better than junior doctors at making diagnoses because they have more experience seeing different presentations of the same illness. We talked about how there are computer programs that are attempting to duplicate this skill. There are also all kinds of "rules" that attempt to identify a specific pattern of disease, but they are all only a poor approximation for the expert doctor.

The key to diagnosis is to take into account the whole picture—something difficult to do for a new trainee or a computer (for different reasons). It's that much more difficult if everyone before you has been focused on another diagnosis. It's a lesson I share with my junior residents and medical students: if something doesn't make sense, start over. Ask the patient to tell the story again. Think through things with fresh eyes. Otherwise, you will miss the diagnosis, just as other doctors before you have.

A second pitfall illustrated in this example is the *end-all-be-all of tests*. Both the primary care doctor and the ER doctor wanted Annette to get a CT scan of her chest because they were concerned about PE. If the test were positive, it would indeed prove to be useful, because it would make the diagnosis: she would have a PE. But they didn't consider what would have happened if the test were negative, or inconclusive, or if she had another incidental finding like the lung nodule. They also didn't consider what *else* could be causing her symptoms—which turned out to be something that the CT couldn't have diagnosed.

All tests all have risks and costs associated with them. CT scans come with them a significant risk of radiation. It is estimated that up to 2 percent of all cancers in the United States is attributable to radiation from CT scans.[4] There are other risks, too, such as the risk of allergic reaction to the

IV contrast used in the CT, and the risk of IV contrast causing kidney damage. Even a simple blood draw can cause skin breakdown and infection. Moreover, simple tests often lead to further tests that are more invasive and have other associated harms.[5]

The d-dimer test that the ER doctor ordered illustrates this point well. D-dimer is a molecule that derives from the body's natural ability to break down blood clots. In patients with PE and other serious clotting problems it can be found circulating in the bloodstream at high levels. But d-dimer is not a specific test for PE. In other words, people can have a high level of circulating d-dimer for a variety of reasons ranging from a history of recent surgery or trauma, to other conditions like cancer or infections.

The d-dimer test is meant to be a screening test to reduce the need for the CT scan: if you have a negative d-dimer test, you can avoid the CT. So, one might think that the introduction of this test would have lead to fewer CT scans, right? Wrong! Studies have shown that the advent of the d-dimer testing has resulted in *more*, rather than *fewer* CT scans for PE. That's because the test is nonspecific: that is, you don't have a PE, but the test still screens positive. As a result, the false positives from this "simple blood test" has led to more CTs, which, according to recent studies, has not changed the death rate from PE.[6] (The cynic would add that the increase would have actually led to increased mortality from cancers due to CTs looking for potential PEs.)

The inherent risks of testing are not reason alone to avoid doing the test if the potential benefits make it worthwhile. An unconscious victim of a high-speed car accident may undergo multiple CT scans to make sure there is no fracture in the neck or bleeding in the abdomen—nobody questions the small risk of radiation compared to the very large risk of missing a serious injury. The problem with a cookbook approach to testing is that it leads doctors and patients alike to think about tests as the end result, rather than the process, of making a diagnosis. All that the CT could have told us was whether Annette had a PE. It wouldn't have helped make a further diagnosis.

Ironically, in Annette's case, there was a test that could have been ordered but did not get considered. A sleep study would have been cheap, noninvasive, and easy to conduct. Annette stayed at the hospital for five days and she was already hooked up to monitors. Had she gotten a sleep

---

✚ 911 ACTION TIP

Beware when you are told you must get a test. Make sure you have a discussion with your doctor about this. Ask what the test is intended to show. Will it confirm a diagnosis? If not, is there another test you should get instead?

---

evaluation, her diagnosis of OSA could have been made and she could have commenced treatment months earlier—and avoided months of agony and excessive testing. Of course, a diagnosis of OSA would have to have been suspected in the first place, and that couldn't happen without taking time to listen to her history and making an effort to put together her clinical picture. We make this point about the sleep study to emphasize that we are not opposed to tests; we just want to be sure that we are ordering the right ones, for the right reasons.

What else went wrong in this case? Annette will tell us. Of all the many primary care doctors, ER doctors, and specialists who saw her, nobody really listened to her. Another pitfall in her case is thus *not understanding the story.* A full history involves careful consideration of the sequence of events. In this case, the main theme of Annette's narrative was fatigue: daytime sleepiness that had gotten progressively worse over weeks to months, culminating in her almost crashing her car with her children in it. That was her major concern, and in fact, if you had to assign her a chief complaint, it would have been "tiredness." A PE might manifest in a lot of different ways, but as daytime sleepiness? And the gradual onset of symptoms over weeks also doesn't fit the picture of PE. The doctors who saw her should have asked, Does the diagnosis make sense? Does it explain the patient's symptoms? Did I even understand her story?[7]

The answer should have been no fairly early on. As a result, the pitfall of *not matching the diagnosis to the story* was inevitable. After listening to Annette's story, her doctor could reasonably consider a whole range of possible diagnoses—the **differential diagnosis** (we will talk more about this subject in Chapter 7). In this case, the doctor could be thinking, could she have

---

✚ 911 ACTION TIP

Beware when the diagnosis doesn't make sense to you. Help your doctor perform this common sense check: ask him whether your story fits with the diagnosis. Do all your symptoms make sense in relation to the diagnosis? How does he explain the ones that don't?

---

some sort of infection, like a virus? Well, she did have a cough at one point (so do a lot of people!), and viral illnesses can make you feel tired. However, the onset of her symptoms was weeks ago, and most viral infections don't last that long. Could she have anemia? Potentially, but why? She didn't mention anything about heavy menstrual periods, and she didn't really look pale, but it would be easy enough to check her blood counts. What about a thyroid problem? If her thyroid hormone was low it could account for her weight gain and her fatigue. With a simple blood test, one could check her hormone levels, if that was really the doctor's suspicion. Could it be a medication that she's on? She wasn't prescribed anything except for her asthma inhalers, but maybe she had started taking a new herbal supplement? One would have to ask.

All those considerations would have been reasonable, but at the end of the day, what her doctor should have seen was an obese woman who slept fitfully and could hardly stay awake during the day. Her sister tells her she's snoring. At this point, sleep apnea should be at or near the *top* of the list of diagnoses. Working through a diagnosis requires thinking about how to best explain the whole story.

There is one final, but very important, pitfall here: *not addressing the patient's primary concern.* Annette was mainly worried about being tired all the time. In her narrative, it was clear that the concern about falling asleep while driving was what prompted her to seek medical care. Yet, she didn't feel like her doctor heard her—and she was right. Analyses of patient-physician interactions have shown that the patient's main concern is not elicited 37 percent of the time.[8] If the doctors had paid closer attention to that part of the history, perhaps the entire story would have come together very differently.

✚ 911 ACTION TIP

If your primary concern was not addressed make sure to bring it up again. "But the main reason I came in was to talk about my [tiredness, headache, shortness of breath, etc.]. Can you explain what's been causing this?" Hold your doctor accountable for answering this basic question—after all, it's why you went to her in the first place.

✚ 911 ACTION TIP

Always tell your doctor exactly what medications you are taking. If you stopped taking a medication, explain why. Is it because it was too expensive, in which case perhaps you can get a cheaper alternative? Is it because there were side effects, in which case your doctor can try something else?

Dr. Wen: There's just one more thing I want to emphasize before we leave Annette's story. Remember how Annette tells us that her primary doctor gave her a prescription and she didn't fill it, but that she couldn't tell this to her doctor? It took me years to figure out that I had to ask, really ask, to find out if my patients were taking their medications as prescribed. Patients are afraid to disappoint their doctors. They may not want to tell their doctor their real reason for not taking the medication. I've seen doctors give this one asthmatic child heaps of drugs because they thought nothing was working, but it was actually that the parents never filled any prescriptions because they couldn't afford it. I've seen diabetic patients come in with seizures from really low blood sugar because their doctor increased their insulin dose, without realizing that the reason the previous dose didn't work was because they weren't taking their medications right. I've seen an elderly woman who everyone thought had impossible-to-control blood pressures be fine on medication when her doctors figured out that she wasn't taking any of her pills because her eyesight was going and she couldn't read the instructions. Doctors should try to figure out if their patients are taking the medications they prescribed, but I also encourage patients to tell their doctors the truth.

✚ 911 ACTION TIP

Always answer your doctor's questions honestly. You must be totally straightforward with your doctor, and you should expect your doctor to be just as frank and open with you. If you are worried about your doctor's response, consider prefacing your statement. "I know we talked about quitting smoking last time, but doctor, I want to be honest with you—I haven't been able to quit yet."

Dr. Kosowsky: Being perfectly honest applies to other matters, too. I've found that patients have all kinds of reasons to not tell the truth. Maybe you don't want to tell your doctor that you're still smoking, or how much alcohol you're drinking, because you're embarrassed. But this could make a difference in how your disease is presenting. Maybe you want a second opinion but don't want to offend your doctor, so you don't mention that you actually already had a CT scan somewhere else last week. But this could increase your risks from a repeat CT scan. Ultimately, you need to be very honest. It really could be a matter of life or death.

Annette: After they made my diagnosis of OSA and I got a sleeping mask to wear at night, I've felt like a new person. I'm not tired during the day, at least not any more tired than you would expect a mother of two young kids to be! I don't worry about falling asleep at the wheel anymore, not even close. My biggest issue is trying to lose the weight, and that's still hard as always.

What's my thought on the way things went? Well, I wish the diagnosis had been made earlier and everyone hadn't been so fixated on a blood clot. My lesson for patients is to ask your doctors how all the symptoms you have fit into their thought process. If I had asked that earlier, they probably could have seen that the blood clot theory didn't make sense and that they should have looked elsewhere.

911 REVIEW

- Help your doctors avoid these pitfalls of cookbook medicine: diagnostic momentum, end-all-be-all of tests, and not understanding the whole story.
- If you are told you must get a test, ask for a discussion with your doctor.
- Tell your doctor what you are really concerned about. Make sure that it is addressed before you leave the office.

Five

The College Student with a Bad Headache

The next story comes from a major teaching hospital in Boston. Recall that there are both resident physicians and attending physicians (along with nurses, techs, and so forth) who provide clinical care in teaching hospitals. This example of cookbook medicine illustrates how differences of opinion can play out among practitioners.

Danielle La Conte is a twenty-year-old college student at the New England Conservatory. She started playing the violin when she was three and had always dreamed about being a concert violinist. When she entered full-time music study, though, she started to realize that it wasn't realistic. This wasn't too much of a disappointment for her; since her chamber music trio toured the Middle East last summer, she's been intrigued by international relations. The field seems suited to her personality, she says, because she loves different cultures and is the perennial peacemaker among her friends.

Today, Danielle comes to the ER with a headache. When she woke up this morning, her head hurt badly. Her mouth was dry, and when she tried to get up to go to the bathroom, she felt like she was getting faint.

She attributed all of this to drinking too much the night before—normally she has one or two drinks when she's out with friends; last night, it was one of her roommate's birthday, and she did three or four shots and had a few beers on top of that.

"The last time I had a hangover was a couple of years ago, and I think this was how I felt then," she says. "My roommate Jackie told me to drink lots of water."

Throughout the day, she felt too nauseous to eat or drink. When the headache didn't go away in the afternoon, she called her mother. Her mom convinced her to go to the ER to make sure everything was OK.

Triage nurse: I see this young girl who tells me that she's having a bad headache after drinking last night. She doesn't have a fever. The only thing abnormal about her vital signs is that when she stands up, her heart rate speeds up. That's a sign of dehydration. She says her headache is a 10 out of 10, but I see her there in the waiting room, chatting away on her cell phone with a magazine open on her lap, so how bad can her headache be, right?

I figure she needs to get some treatment for her headache, probably some fluids for her dehydration and some Tylenol, so I send her to the Fast Track area. That's the same area we put coughs and colds and minor injuries, because the treatment is simple and then patients are on their way.

Nurse in Fast Track: I see that the triage nurse had written "10/10 headache." I ask her more about her headaches, and she tells me she's had headaches before, but this is different. She doesn't say why or how, but it's just different. And she says that this morning, she just woke up with a pounding headache and then threw up.

Danielle: Yeah, I tried to eat and then I threw up. I think it happened to me last time when I drank too much. That's what my other roommate Mary Ellen says happens the morning after when you have a hangover, too. I didn't think it was that big of a deal. But then all these doctors start coming in and getting me scared.

Attending: The nurse approaches me and my resident and tells us we should come see this patient. She describes a young girl who woke up and developed a headache—worse than she ever had in her life—with a fairly sudden onset. And has been vomiting. As far as I'm concerned, that's a classic story for a subarachnoid hemorrhage—a rare, but very serious type of bleeding into the brain.

Resident: I go to see Danielle. As I talk with her, I begin to feel more reassured. Danielle says to me that she has had headaches before, that this is a little different but not that different, and that she'd been partying pretty heavily last night. She tells me that she woke up with the headache, vomited twice, and hasn't felt like eating or drinking anything all day.

It's been a few years since I was in college, but I haven't forgotten what a hangover feels like. I attribute the nausea and vomiting to her hangover, and the headache, at least in part, to dehydration, so I order her symptomatic treatment: IV fluids, Tylenol, and medication for nausea. I don't think it's likely that this is a stroke or bleeding in the brain because her story is so consistent with a hangover.

Attending: Attendings have to see every patient who comes through the ER, and ultimately we are the ones responsible for the medical decision-making. In this case, I disagree with the resident. A subarachnoid hemorrhage is no joke. It's a life-threatening diagnosis. One of the hallmarks is "worst headache of your life," which the patient does not deny when I ask her directly. She rates her pain 10 on a scale of 10. That's pretty high. The pain scale is a subjective method for measuring pain, and she's talking to me normally, not like she really has the worst headache of her life (and we'd seen her text on her phone)—but still, it's documented that her headache is 10 out of 10. Since brain bleed is a "can't miss" diagnosis for doctors, we have to "rule it out."

Danielle: I get a needle in my arm and they give me some fluids and some medications for nausea that really help. After half an hour or so, my nausea's completely gone and my headache's down to about a 3 out of 10. Like I wouldn't even have noticed it if someone didn't ask me about it. But they tell me I might have bleeding in my brain. I can't believe it. How did that happen? I think I was drunk last night but not that drunk. I didn't fall or anything. I've always imagined that people with a brain hemorrhage would be really sick—unconscious or in a coma. That's pretty scary stuff! They tell me they need a CT scan of my head, so of course I said yes.

Resident: The head CT scan is negative. You would think this is good news, and yes, it is, but have we really "ruled out" a subarachnoid hemorrhage? Head CTs can miss up to 5 percent of all subarachnoid hemorrhages,[1] so the textbooks say that if you suspect a bleed and the CT is negative, you have to do another test: a spinal tap.

The question I have is this: do we really suspect bleeding in the brain? And if it's not a bleed, what else, if anything, do we need to be worried about? By now, Danielle is feeling much better. She's on the phone with her friends making dinner plans. She asks me if she can go because she has a music rehearsal session in an hour, and she wants to shower and change before that so she can go out tonight. Admittedly, I haven't seen more than a couple dozen patients with a true subarachnoid hemorrhage, but this really doesn't fit the picture of someone who is having a serious bleeding in the brain.

Nurse: The whole thing is getting ridiculous. Yeah, I was worried when I first heard the story. But then it changed. I talked with her two roommates over the phone and they confirmed her story, that the onset of the headaches was not sudden and this same thing happened when she got really drunk a few years ago. Now, it seems clear that the girl has a hangover. If I had a hangover, I wouldn't want a head CT or, God forbid, a spinal tap.

I tell all my girlfriends, stay out of the ER if you have a hangover, 'cause I know what they would want to do. The docs, they always want to "rule out" this or "rule out" that because they're so worried about getting sued.

Attending: Do I really suspect that the patient is having a bleeding in the brain? No, I don't. It was very unlikely to begin with and I think it's even more unlikely after the head CT came back negative. But making sure it's *not* a head bleed is the standard of care. If we want to rule out a subarachnoid hemorrhage, we get a head CT; if that's negative, then a lumbar puncture. That's the pathway we follow.

You'll get burned if you don't follow this pathway. A couple of years back, I had a case where I missed a subarachnoid on a young woman—the resident and I didn't think she could have had it, so we sent her home without any studies. She came back the next day in a coma. In looking back, the problem was that we should have taken a better history—it would have been pretty clear what the problem was because all the warning signs were there. But I just can't afford to miss this kind of diagnosis again.

In this case, I can see that the resident isn't as keen to follow this pathway, so I tell her that if she doesn't want to talk to the patient about the spinal tap, I'll do it.

Resident: When my attending put it like that, it was hard to argue. His point is that this is the subarachnoid algorithm we're following, so if we get one test, we need to do the other part of it, too. What I don't understand is how our patient is on the "subarachnoid pathway" if it's not the most likely diagnosis by a long shot. Also, is it true that once we're on the pathway, there's no way to get off? It seems bizarre that if we do one test, we are obligated to do another. I actually want to send her home. Nevertheless, the attending has the final say, so I follow his lead and tell the patient why we need to do this lumbar puncture.

Danielle: A spinal tap? When they first tell me, I think it's a bad joke. I've never heard of anyone who got a spinal tap. It sounds really painful. The resident tells me one of the common side effects is that some people experience a *worse* headache after the procedure. So what's the point of that when I've gotten rid of my headache? I really don't want to do it.

Actually, my friends are already on the way to pick me up for rehearsal because I thought I would get to go. I get dressed. Then the older doctor comes in and says if I don't get the spinal tap, I'll have to sign something saying I'm leaving against medical advice and my insurance may not pay for this ER visit. I can't believe it! At this point, my roommate Mary Ellen is there, too, and she swears up and down that we had a lot to drink last night and that my headache this morning wasn't that bad. I phone my mother to talk to her, then the doctor asks to speak with her. He gets on the phone with her and tells her I need it. My mom freaks out and says she's driving from Cincinnati to see me. I feel like my hands are tied.

Nurse: They all get ready to do the lumbar puncture and have the gowns and needles and everything open. The resident is in there getting the needles and tubes ready. Danielle says she has to go to the bathroom. She goes out, and never comes back. She leaves all her clothes and shoes, and runs out in her hospital gown! I think she knew best, to just get the heck outta there when she had a chance.

Resident: I can totally understand why she ran away; she's young and she got scared, and she didn't want to do a procedure that she didn't really need. The unfortunate thing about her leaving like that is that she never got her discharge instructions. I wish I could have told her what she should expect and what warning signs to watch out for. If she does have a hangover, she should continue to feel better. On the other hand, if she starts having a worse headache, if she starts vomiting again, if she gets more sleepy, she should come back to the ER. She's a reliable person and I would have trusted that she would follow my instructions. She lives with two girls who could watch her closely and make sure she was OK. Instead, now she will probably do anything to avoid coming back. We scared her so much that if anything were to happen, she probably won't seek medical care.

Attending: We probably could have approached the whole situation better. At the very least, we should have had her fill out the "against medical advice" form.[2] I instructed my resident on what to do next: write down everything. We offered the patient the procedure and explained the importance of ruling out a hemorrhage; she refused. I stick by our original decision: we managed this patient correctly by going down the subarachnoid pathway.

Danielle's case exemplifies several recognizable pitfalls that we saw in Jerry's and Annette's stories. The fixation on "ruling out" a subarachnoid hemorrhage is the pitfall we know well by now as *worst-case reasoning*. The fast-paced nature of ER work, the high acuity of patient population, and fear of litigation make ER doctors particularly vulnerable to worst-case thinking. Other specialties are not immune; this is a universal problem in medicine today. We saw how Annette Golding's internist was fixated on the diagnosis of pulmonary embolism. Had Danielle gone to her primary care doctor, she might have received a referral slip to get a head CT in the ER. Thinking about the worst case may be important, but "ruling out" should not exclusively drive doctors' thinking, especially when there are more likely diagnoses.

Similarly, just like adhering to the *path always followed* for PE means d-dimer and then CT scan, following the "pathway" for subarachnoid hemorrhage lead doctors to do a head CT, then lumbar puncture. Once the pathway was initiated, it seemed that there was no way to exit the pathway— not even when the patient was so against it and the suspicion was extremely low. But this is the kind of blind adherence that is reflexive, rather than reflective. A more thoughtful approach would involve considering the range of possible diagnoses, weighing the pros and cons of confirmatory tests, and continually reassessing the situation, together with the patient.

In Danielle's case, the situation did evolve, but the diagnostic approach never changed. This is another diagnostic pitfall of cookbook medicine: *not being able to adjust to change.* It's possible that Danielle told different providers slightly different stories, or at least that different people understood different things from what she told them. The triage nurse heard a story consistent with hangover, whereas the second nurse was worried about a head bleed. Once this worst-case scenario potential diagnosis got voiced, the attending stuck with it, despite it not fitting with the story that he and the resident obtained. The attending stuck with it even after Danielle's roommate came in and corroborated Danielle's story. That Danielle's symptoms improved and that her head CT was negative should have further steered the diagnosis away from subarachnoid hemorrhage. The underlying problem is that cookbook recipes, pathways, and algorithms are, by definition, inflexible; a very different result would have come about if the diagnosis were individualized to Danielle in the first place.

The devil's advocate would point out that the attending may not be wrong and, in fact, that doctors can rarely be 100 percent certain of a diagnosis based on history alone. Does erring on the side of caution make sense in an acute situation when the patient's story may not be clear? Absolutely.

✚ 911 ACTION TIP

Beware that your doctor may not be willing to adjust his initial plan. As test results come in or other new information comes up, ask your doctor how it changes his approach for you. Let your doctor know how you feel after a specific treatment, and ask him if this response changes his thinking about your diagnosis.

✚ 911 ACTION TIP

Beware when you get different reactions from different members of your healthcare team. For example when your doctor is responding to a particular aspect of your story with a lot of concern when your nurse isn't. Ask your doctor or nurse why this is the case. Did someone misunderstand something you said? The earlier you can correct a misunderstanding, the better.

However, as the clinical situation evolves and more is known, the likelihood of any particular diagnosis changes, and the diagnostic approach must be adjusted accordingly—a process that does not occur in cookbook medicine.

Dr. Kosowsky: It's not infrequent that my resident and I will hear somewhat different stories from the same patient. I don't necessarily presume that I am right and the resident is wrong. Or if it's a nurse, that I'm right and the nurse is wrong. What often helps is that we all come together to the room and have the patient clarify it together for us. We usually find that someone misinterpreted something that was said, or that the patient forgot to tell one of us a piece of the story. This is normal, even expected; it's nearly impossible to tell exactly the same story to two, sometimes three or more, different people! So clarification in the form of a huddle is necessary for good communication and good patient care.

A further pitfall represented in Danielle's case is that of *anecdote-based practice*. This is the opposite of evidence-based practice. Now, we also have criticisms of evidence-based practice, particularly as applied to diagnosis and irrational adherence to algorithms—it's part of the reason we are stuck with cookbook medicine. But the opposite extreme should be avoided, too. When the attending points to a single missed case of subarachnoid hemorrhage driving his thought process, he's falling into this trap of anecdote-based practice. However frightening his previous experience was, allowing an isolated case to drive one's overall practice pattern is not good medicine.[3]

Dr. Wen: I attended a Mortality & Morbidity conference a few weeks ago where they discussed a case of a missed subarachnoid hemorrhage. This was a young woman who ate what she thought was bad Chinese food and had profuse vomiting. The ER thought she was fine, maybe had food poisoning or a viral syndrome, and sent her home. She came back the next day with more vomiting and this time, they found she had a subarachnoid hemorrhage.

We all got really scared after this presentation. A lot of us started doing more CT scans and lumbar punctures just to be sure. It wasn't as if new research came out saying that we should be doing more scans or that our index of suspicion wasn't high enough. It was this one case driving our practice. This may be a human response, but it would be even more instructive to use anecdotes as opportunities to look for patterns and learn lessons, rather than to develop a new "rule."[4]

All's well that ends well. Danielle never came back to the ER, but she did get in touch with the resident (who was Dr. Wen) through a mutual friend: she wanted to ask about study-abroad scholarship programs in the U.K. At the time of this writing, Danielle is applying to a master's in Peace Studies in Ireland. She has no particular love for the ER, and her advice is to stay far away unless you have something seriously wrong.

"And be prepared to run away if you don't agree with what they're offering," she adds.

That's not the lesson we hope you will take away, but we do think there is a lot to be learned from Danielle's experience. Cookbook medicine leads practitioners to believe that there is one way to do things: by a set "pathway" and by that one pathway only. As a result, practitioners tend to present dichotomous, either-or options to patients. Danielle was told that if she refused the spinal tap, she would have to sign out against medical advice. Had Jerry, with his pulled muscle, told his doctor that he didn't want to spend the night, he probably would have been asked to do the same. They would have been trapped—literally—by the doctors and nurses, by the hospital, and by the medical system.

We do not believe such an approach is conducive to good patient care. As in other parts of life, most decisions in medicine are not so clear-cut with choices that are absolutely right or wrong. Refusing a spinal tap might be a reasonable decision in this or other scenarios, and that decision should be respected as a basic expression of patient autonomy.[5] We believe in a partnership approach where decisions are made together, not simply based on worst-case thinking or adherence to a depersonalized recipe.

911 REVIEW

- Cookbook medicine can literally make patients feel trapped.
- Members of your healthcare team may understand your story differently. Find out why, and correct mistakes early.
- A fatal flaw of cookbook medicine is the inability to adapt to change. By definition, pathways and recipes are inflexible, while you, the patient, are dynamic.

Six

The Woman Who Fainted at the Sight of a Sandwich

May Gillespie has a story to tell and she will not stop until she tells it. That's the way she's always been. "My mom says I've been an activist ever since I stood up to this big second-grader who stole all the kindergarten kids' treats. That was half a century ago!"

Indeed, May came of age in the 1970s and made a career out of her activism. Even while raising her four kids and running her own business as founder and owner of an independent bookstore, she was a volunteer lobbyist for NOW and a peer counselor for Planned Parenthood. She helped to start a local school for pregnant teens that allows them continue their education and then assists them to find jobs.

"I'm so much a child of my generation that I'm almost a caricature of myself," she likes to say.

As a recent divorcée with her youngest child in college, May had more time on her hands than she ever had before. A group of women from her town formed an exercise club, and May found herself joining the neighborhood gym—a women's only gym—with them. She loves to talk and this was another social outlet to see her friends. To her pleasant surprise, she liked the gym and the way that exercise was making her feel.

"Sure, I was sore, but I felt better than I had for a long time," she said. Soon, she and her friends Joanna and Susan—also recently divorced empty-nesters—got into the habit of working out every other day at the gym, doing about forty minutes on the elliptical machine followed by an hour-long yoga class.

A couple of months or so into her new routine, May began feeling a bit under the weather. Over the weekend, her stomach had been upset and she didn't have much of an appetite. She didn't make much of it: a number of the women in the exercise group had come down with a stomach bug, and there was something going around at her school as well.

Hoping to battle through whatever it was, she decided she would go to the gym Monday morning, despite feeling too sick to eat much for breakfast. When Joanna and Susan came to pick her up, they noticed that she wasn't her usual self, notwithstanding her protestations that she was "just fine." At the gym, May started on the elliptical machine. She was much quieter than usual; she was really needing all her energy to work out. All her muscles ached, and she was gasping for breath. Still, she tried to make small talk to take her mind off her queasy stomach; she was hoping no one would notice.

But her friends could tell something was up. "Maybe we should all break early and head for the sauna," one of them suggested. Joanna had tried using the hot tub after a workout last week and it had really relaxed her. Maybe it would help clear her head, May thought, as the women headed for the sauna.

The hot steam did feel good, but May soon found the humid air to be too stifling. So she stood up. Or, more precisely, she tried to stand up. Almost immediately, she felt light-headed. There were bright spots dancing in front of her eyes. Sweat pored down her face

She slumped to the ground on her knees. Someone screamed. People were at her side immediately; they sounded far away to her. Joanna and Susan helped her to the locker room, where she managed to pull on her jacket to get ready to leave.

"Are you sure you don't want us to bring you to the doctor?" Susan asked.

"I'll be fine," May said. "Why don't you just drop me off at home? The two of you can go for lunch without me." Funny, she liked to help other people, but hated getting help herself. And the last thing she wanted was to go to a hospital.

"You really should have something to eat, dear." May shook her head.

"Come on," Joanna urged. "At least it'll make *us* feel better."

May groaned. Joanna carried food with her everywhere, and she thrust what looked like a half-eaten tuna sandwich in front of her.

Ugh! Rotten fish, how disgusting! Those were the last thoughts May had inside the gym. The next thing she remembered, she was on a stretcher being hoisted into an ambulance.

Triage Nurse: By the time the paramedics give their report, we all have a pretty good idea about what happened. This lady wasn't feeling well; she hadn't eaten anything all day; she went into a sauna and had a "vasovagal reaction." That's what happens when you faint: you get light-headed, you see spots, you have a low blood pressure, and you pass out.

Doctor: When I first see this woman, she's in no real distress, as far as I can tell. It's a decent story for a simple fainting spell. But I have to be worried about her heart. She's postmenopausal and she probably has borderline diabetes and hypertension and high cholesterol—all the classic risk factors for heart disease. And there are other things that have be "ruled out" in terms of why she passed out.

But I can't even begin to sort out these issues. That's because she has what I call the "positive review of systems." This is one talkative lady with a bad case of verbal diarrhea. First she wants to convince me to join some crazy left-wing group and donate money to this friend running for city council—not in Boston but somewhere in Arizona. I tell her I don't have time and start asking questions, but she just seems incapable of answering anything. She says yes to anything I ask. Headache? Yes. Chest pain? Yes. I mean, . . . I think so. Which part of the chest are you asking about? Do you think I'm having a heart attack? Palpitations? Like when your heart skips a beat? Oh yes, definitely. I had some today, stomach pain? Well, not really pain, but yes. It could just be a stomach virus. Of course, I haven't really eaten that much in the past couple of days, so . . . and on and on like that.

When faced with difficult patients like this who have a whole constellation of symptoms and an impossible story, I've learned to just focus on one symptom—the one that's likely to be the most serious. In her case, I was already worried about her heart, so I decide that she falls into the "rule-out cardiac syncope pathway," meaning that we are going to focus on her heart as the reason for her passing out.

Medical Student: I could see that the doctors and nurses weren't terribly excited about this patient. She probably didn't have anything serious, yet she answers yes to everything and kinda just blabbers on. So as the lowly medical student, the rookie member of the team, I get sent to ask her some more questions.

No question this lady is a talker. I find her entertaining. She's one of those typical Cambridge types, you know, the Wellesley grad-turned-hippie-mom-who-gets-into-everyone's-business? Who's super well-meaning but is just loud and talks forever? Anyway, after listening to her for half an hour, the gist of it is that she thinks she had some kind of virus, maybe a stomach bug or something because she's been having vague abdominal pain and nausea for a few days, then today she was at the gym and felt light-headed, then passed out.

Before I can sort out the whole story, the attending doctor comes in and tells us that we're done. There are so many potential things wrong with her; he says we just have to pick one of her complaints and make that the chief complaint, or else we'll never get anywhere.

Doctor: I don't mean that we should ignore everything else about her but one symptom. But here's the bottom line: are we going to send this patient home, or is she going to be admitted to the hospital? There's no debate, right? She has to be admitted, at the very least overnight, for monitoring of her heart rhythm and vital signs, measurement of her cardiac enzymes, and maybe a stress test or ultrasound of her heart in the morning to make sure she doesn't have heart damage. The other stuff, like whether her sinuses are congested or she has diarrhea can be figured out later. We don't have to make a diagnosis; we just have to rule out really bad things and then decide where she's going.

May: I know I'm a talker, and maybe I wasn't being helpful. I just think when someone asks me a question I should answer it honestly. So if someone says, so, how have you been feeling recently, I should tell them how I'm feeling! But all they want to do is talk about my heart. I'm not so sure it's the problem. It was my stomach that didn't feel right. Nobody wants to hear that, though.

ER nurse: There was something about her that didn't look quite like our other "rule-out cardiac syncope" patients. A little while after she gets here, she has the chills, so I go back and check her temperature. It's 100.8. I remember the doctor said something about a virus, and when I tell him about the temperature, he orders some Tylenol for her. The med student does a flu swab and a strep test and these are negative. Four hours after she arrives, she has a bed on the cardiology floor, so she goes from us to there for further evaluation.

May's story doesn't end quite yet. She continued to feel feverish and was nauseated all night. She asked the nurse if she could get any medicine for her stomach pain and she was given some more Tylenol. The next morning she was told that her "cardiac workup" was negative so far and that she just needed to stay for a stress test. Really? She honestly couldn't imagine getting on a treadmill in her condition. She's fine, it's just a virus, the doctors reasoned, and they gave her fluids through the IV. Throughout the day, she couldn't eat or drink.

By the following morning, her temperature had climbed to 102.5. Laboratory tests at that time showed a slight elevation of her liver enzymes, and her belly pain got worse, so that afternoon, a full forty-eight hours after she arrived in the ER, the doctors scheduled for her to get a CT scan of her abdomen.

When the techs arrived to take May for her CT scan, she was having full body rigors and shaking. Her sheets were soaked through. Her heart rate climbed to the 140s—double the normal range—and her blood pressure became dangerously low. Her doctors were paged STAT. Upon reexamining her, they discovered that while all of her cardiac tests had been totally normal, her abdomen was now as rigid as a board.

May's cardiologists consulted the surgery team, who decided to take her to the operating room. They suspected that she had a serious infection in her abdomen. What they found in surgery was that her gallbladder had become gangrenous. It was so infected that it literally died and was producing pus—then burst its infected contents throughout May's abdominal cavity. A large incision was made so that her abdomen could be washed out and rid of all the infected material.

Had her gallbladder infection been discovered when she first went to the hospital, she might have been put on antibiotics two days earlier and gone through a routine procedure to remove the gallbladder. Now instead of a one-hour operation, May was in the operating room for over six hours. Her blood pressure remained low after the operation due to the overwhelming infection and she had to stay in the surgical ICU for three days. The breathing tube was removed but then had to be put back because she was drowsy from all the anesthetics and couldn't breathe on her own. Instead of having an indiscernible scar from a minor operation, May now sports a large twelve-inch scar.

May: Pardon the expression: I felt like crap. After the operation, it took me months to get back on my feet. The thing is, I knew something was wrong all along. The EKGs, the blood tests—they all didn't show anything, but if they'd only asked me about it, I could have told them from the moment I arrived that I had something wrong with my stomach.

Still, I'm one of the lucky ones. I know people who had bad infections and died, and I came out of this OK. I just wish that the doctors had listened a little more to me in the first place and did a more careful evaluation. Maybe they could have caught the gallbladder thing before it got so bad.

In the last chapter, we made reference to the M&M, the Mortality & Morbidity conference that takes place at our hospital and hospitals around the country. May Gillespie's case could have very well been presented at one of these conferences. Thankfully, there was no *mortality*; May recovered after her operation and was able to resume her normal activities. But there was *morbidity*: she went through several uncomfortable days in pain and not knowing what was going on before her diagnosis was made; she had a prolonged and complicated surgical course; and, as a result of the extensive surgery, May not only has a large scar across her belly, but is also likely to have scarring internally that could lead to complications down the road such as bowel obstructions and recurrent infections.

The purpose of M&M is to point out errors made in a particular case that can serve as lessons for others. In a typical M&M, the presenter goes over the case and then an analysis of the errors and suggestions for future improvement. Medical errors can be divided into two categories: system errors and cognitive errors. System errors occur when it is not an individual, but the process itself, that is at fault: for example, if an abnormal lab result is not logged due to a computer system glitch, or if there is a breakdown in communication between doctor and nurse. Cognitive errors, on the other hand, are defects in the thought process of the care providers; many cognitive errors are really just pitfalls of cookbook medicine.[1]

One type of cognitive error made by the doctors early on in this case is the pitfall of *premature closure*. Although the attending acknowledged that there could be many reasons why May fainted, he decided to focus on one—the heart. He reasoned (incorrectly) that the specific diagnosis wouldn't effect his management, since May would have to stay in the hospital overnight anyway. So why bother figuring out an exact cause of her symptoms?

Some of our physician colleagues would say that getting a diagnosis is not the goal of emergency care, that the ER is for making sure there is no life-threatening illness. We do not agree. Getting to a diagnosis is the key to everything else that follows—without a diagnosis, how can treatment be started? How can the patient begin to understand what she has? In this case,

---

✚ 911 ACTION TIP

Beware if your doctor is focused on one system only. If you have several symptoms, but she keeps on going back to one, ask her if she can explain the other symptoms, too. If she tells you she wants to "rule out" something that can explain only one of your symptoms, ask, "Is there anything else this could be? How do you make sense of my other symptoms?" You can make sure that premature closure does not happen.

focusing on the "workup" of one particular system (in this case the heart) led to a delay in life-saving treatment. Even if it didn't, why have the patient suffer and be anxious rather than identifying the definitive diagnosis early on? This is perhaps even more important for patients who are discharged from the ER, because this will often be their only encounter with a doctor for that problem.

Another pitfall in May's case is one that we mentioned before, that of *diagnostic momentum.* The initial doctor in this case was not focused on the diagnostic process because he figured May would have to stay in the hospital anyway. He settled on "rule-out cardiac syncope" only because it seemed consistent with someone who fainted. May thus ended up on a cardiology floor to "work up" her supposed heart problem. Subsequent doctors took their cue from the first doctor and failed to connect the dots until May became very sick from her infected gallbladder. In this case, May was lucky (as she acknowledges) because even though her blood pressure dropped and her fever became very high, she had enough reserve to make it through this episode. Another patient may not have been so lucky, and premature closure and accompanying diagnostic momentum could have easily led to other "M" in M&M.

These concepts closely associate with another problem we alluded to before: *fitting the presentation to the recipe rather than the patient.* May started out with a very broad list (the differential diagnosis) for what could be causing her symptoms. The moment the doctor started to hone in on the "cardiac" issues, the recipe became all about the heart: the heart enzymes, the treadmill test, etc. Once the pathway got set, it became very difficult to change horses in midstream and think about the patient's presentation in a broader context. Better yet to make sure your doctor does not use any recipe, and help him maintain an open mind.

✚ 911 ACTION TIP

Even if you feel like you've been headed down a pathway for a while, it's never too late to ask why. Asking the question may be the impetus your doctor needs to think about the appropriateness of the pathway for you.

Then there's the matter of the patient herself. May is what some would call "*a difficult patient.*" With cookbook medicine, there is a tendency to blame the patient if their symptoms don't fit into a set recipe. Take the patient who says she "just doesn't feel well" or "hurts all over"—unless someone comes up with an algorithm for these things (which is unlikely!), the cookbook doctor is going to be stuck. Equally troubling is the patient who fits into too many algorithms: chest pain when she breathes and worst headache of her life with numbness in an arm: which pathway does one choose? One option would be to select "all of the above," but even the most committed proponent of cookbook diagnosis has to feel a little bit foolish ordering a slew of tests without any direction at all. We're talking the ultimate shotgun approach.

Dr. Kosowsky: I get asked by residents and students all the time what to do if I have a difficult historian. By that they usually mean someone who has trouble giving a consistent history, who may ramble on and tell you ten things are wrong with them along with their life history and their cat's and dog's histories, too.

I give these students a reply they don't want to hear, because I tell them that there's no such thing as a difficult historian, only a bad history-taker. A lot of times these patients have long stories because there really is a lot going on. Someone who's had complicated heart problems for thirty-five years has a lot of ground to cover. Many conditions are not just defined by one symptom, but by a whole constellation of them. Also, sometimes the rambling history is itself a clue: to the patient's state of mind, to their concep-

---

✚ 911 ACTION TIP

Doctors may complain about the "difficult patients" out there, but just the same, there are "difficult doctors," too. Be on the lookout for doctors who appear to be too busy to listen to your story or who seem defensive when you ask them questions. If you have a choice of doctors, those are the ones to avoid. In Chapter 14, we provide some more tips for spotting the "difficult doctors"—and, if you're stuck with them, for dealing with them.

tion of illness and healing, even to an underlying diagnosis like depression, anxiety, or dementia.

There was a study where researchers audiotaped ER encounters, and found that only 20 percent of patients were able to state their presenting symptoms without interruptions. The average time to interruption was 12 seconds.[2] It's a good illustration of how intolerant doctors can be when it comes to actually listening to their patients. Why is it that they seem to prefer fishing for symptoms that they know how to "work up"? They'll hear a patient talking about dizziness or weakness, or "just not feeling right" and then they'll interrupt a patient and begin to ask about other symptoms. Shortness of breath? No, OK. Abdominal pain? No, OK. Chest pain? Yes? Why? Because now they have something to put into an algorithm. Meanwhile, they've missed the opportunity to get the real story.

Dr. Wen: When I first learned about Josh's method of approaching patients, I asked him what he would have done with a patient like this. I can easily see how it seems like May Gillespie with her million symptoms could take a long time to talk to. How can we manage this when we are also seeing ten other patients? What Josh said I took to heart, which is to consider that it's worth it to invest an extra five or ten minutes upfront to avoid long delays, unnecessary tests, and possibly days or weeks of uncertainty for the patient. At the end of the day, it's about the patient. It may not seem efficient to spend time listening to Mrs. Gillespie's life story, but it's even more inefficient to send someone like her to a cardiology service for a surgical emergency. Not to mention it's really just poor patient care to leave the patient without even an attempt at a diagnosis.

A related pitfall to *labeling the patient as the "difficult historian"* is *dismissing the patient's story as a "positive review of systems"*. The **review of systems** is a comprehensive review that the doctor performs as part of a complete medical history, going system by system—respiratory, gastrointestinal, neurologic, and so on—through all the possible symptoms that a patient could have. The idea is to make sure that no symptom, however minor, is missed. It's easy to write off someone like May Gillespie as a completely "positive review of systems" when she answers yes to so many questions.

But many illnesses invariably involve several body systems at once. For example, a simple cold gives you a runny nose and maybe a cough, so the respiratory system is affected. You might also have a headache and muscle aches, too, implicating the both neurological and musculoskeletal systems. In May's case, her gallbladder infection had probably been smoldering for a while, accounting for generalized symptoms like nausea, fatigue, and low-grade fever, in addition to any abdominal discomfort attributable to the gallbladder itself. The fainting spell might have been due to a combination of dehydration and the pain from her infected gallbladder.

May's symptoms neither individually nor collectively fit well into a diagnostic algorithm for fainting, or any other cookbook recipe for that matter. However, taken as a whole, the pattern suggests an infection inside the abdomen. The problem is that when questions are asked in isolation as part of some yes-or-no questioning recipe, they made no sense. In her case, it took doctors days to figure this out. Even after May got sicker, their first inclination was that she was fine, at least from a cardiac standpoint. But how does a chest pain pathway or fainting pathway deal with a patient who has a fever? It takes thinking outside the box—or better yet, not putting the patient in the box to begin with—to assess the whole picture and make a correct diagnosis.

Dr. Kosowsky: I talked to the medical student who saw May initially. I acknowledged that it's sometimes easier to blame the patient when you walk away with a poor history. I told him, though, that as a doctor, it will be his job to elicit the patient's story. Not the story that he wants to hear, but the real story. Learning how to elicit a history takes time and effort and lots of practice; it's the reason it takes so many years to be a doctor, the reason why it's called the "practice" of medicine.

This medical student had the right instinct: he wanted to listen to the patient; he just wasn't sure how. He should be encouraged to keep trying. Similarly, patients should be encouraged to be direct and open and tell their whole stories to their doctors. Hopefully, our book will help empower patients to insist on open communication with their doctors—the kind of open communication that is key to good medical care.

May Gillespie now sports a large scar down the center of her abdomen. She also has a new focus for her activism: patient advocacy. Adding to her list of many other activities, May now volunteers her time as a patient liaison for local Boston hospitals. Her new passion: patient-provider communication.

"Lack of communication was one major reason why I got so sick," May says. "Improving communication is critical, and I believe it has to begin with empowering patients to speak up and to get their doctors to listen."

911 REVIEW

- Focusing on "ruling out" problems rather than figuring out the diagnosis often leads to missed diagnoses, which can result in bad and sometimes fatal outcomes.
- Many diseases present with multiple symptoms. It's important to resist your doctors' efforts to limit your report of multiple symptoms.
- Doctors may think there are difficult patients, but patients should also be aware of the difficult doctor.

Part III

The Building Blocks
to Avoid Misdiagnosis

Dr. Wen: When I first described the concept of our book to my husband, Sebastian, he didn't get it. More precisely, he didn't see what the problem was with medical care today. After all, isn't America supposed to have the best healthcare system in the world?

Just a few months ago, he had an encounter in the ER, that changed his mind. When he was younger, he had some issues with a rapid heart rate. Every once in a while, he would feel as if his heart was "fluttering." Sometimes he would wake up with a feeling like his heart was beating so fast it was going to come out of his chest. It was uncomfortable and at times scary. But the fast rate would inevitably resolve on its own, sometimes with the aid of maneuvers—like holding his breath—that his doctors taught him. He saw a cardiologist for the fast heart rate and was reassured that this was a benign condition. This particular evening, though, he (and I) couldn't get his rapid heart rate to stop. After five hours, he was feeling light-headed (probably from all the breath-holding), so we decided to go to an ER.

What happened next was a predictable sequence of events. He was pegged as a man in his late thirties with "chest discomfort." Never mind that he kept pointing out that his chest was uncomfortable because his heart had been beating at three times the normal rate for hours! He was put on the same "chest pain pathway" that Jerry the mechanic was: blood tests, chest X-ray, the whole nine yards. Even after his fast heart rate resolved (on its own, might I add), he was told he needed to stay overnight for more labs and a treadmill test.

"But I play sports and I run four times a week," Sebastian told them. "Why do I have to stay?"

"Because it's the protocol," he was told. The chest pain pathway was the recipe that had to be followed. He had to do it—or sign out against medical advice.

Dr. Kosowsky: I bet that now, your husband gets what you mean when you talk about cookbook medicine.

Dr. Wen: And not just that—he never wanted to see a doctor ever again! He felt trapped—forced to stay in the hospital against his will.

Dr. Kosowsky: This is why it's important to read on! Now that your husband—and our readers—has seen the failures of cookbook medicine, it's time to take a look at how we can do better.

Dr. Wen: Before we go on, I do want to say one thing: in no way do we mean for our book to be an indictment of doctors. We believe that doctors, by and large, are well intentioned. They went into medicine for the right reasons, and they are trying to do their best. It's the modern system of medical training that drills cookbook recipes into them and trains them to miss diagnoses. Medical practice has gotten further and further away from true patient-centered care. The system has failed all of us, both patients and doctors alike.

Dr. Kosowsky: And this is why it's so important for you, our patients, to be your own advocate. The whole premise of our book is that you have the power to revolutionize your medical care; that what you do really matters, for you and for everyone else.

Dr. Wen: So let's go! In this section, we illustrate the principles and building blocks to help your doctor get to your diagnosis. Our ✚ 911 Action Tips demonstrate how to apply it to your medical care.

Seven

A Crash Course on Diagnosis

There is a mystique about medical education that the public finds fascinating. TV shows highlight the intensity, humor, challenges, and interpersonal conundrums involved in the process of becoming a doctor. If you've watched *Grey's Anatomy* and *ER* or read *House of God*, you probably think you have some idea of what medical training is all about. But do you?

In Chapter 2, we described the process of medical training, from medical student to resident to attending. Now, we take you on a whirlwind tour of what physicians-in-training actually learn in the course of their medical studies. To avoid being misdiagnosed by your doctors, you need to know how doctors are taught to see patients. We illustrate how doctors approach diagnosis: the steps they take in thinking through what might be wrong with their patients. In this chapter, we define key terminology and point out important steps in the diagnostic process—along with where things go wrong and what you can do to remedy it.

Dr. Wen: Growing up, my favorite author was Agatha Christie. How I adored Miss Marple and Hercule Poirot! I loved how they always knew how to ask questions in the right way, with the right nuance, to get at the real answer. I loved how they pieced together multiple subtle clues, while sorting through red herrings, to come up with the whodunit. My favorite novel of hers was

Five Little Pigs. It's remarkable how Poirot solved a murder committed many years ago with just the testimony of witnesses alone, without ever seeing the crime scene. This speaks to the power of narrative and observation of subtle clues. Standardized rules and rote algorithms need not apply!

Dr. Kosowsky: I tell my students that becoming a doctor is a lot like becoming a detective. An aspiring detective starts with the basics, like forensic science and criminal justice, but he also has to begin acquiring real-life experience. At first, that mostly happens vicariously. How did the expert detective solve that case? What were the important clues and how were they found? What were they looking for and why? There are a lot of basics in medicine, too: biochemistry, anatomy, physiology. Some people have likened medical training to learning a whole new vocabulary; I think it's more like learning a whole new way to think and process information.

Dr. Wen: That's why we want to take you through the process and explain what medical students learn and how. Curricula vary somewhat among various medical schools, but as we saw in Chapter 2, it's generally divided into first and second year as the "preclinical" years, and then third and fourth year as the "clinical" years. The preclinical time is about classroom learning of some core concepts. One of the first classes students across the country have is **anatomy,** which talks about what goes where in the body. It's pretty clear why this is important.

Anatomy was a pretty big initiation rite for all of us. Our class was divided into groups of four—that is, four to a cadaver. It was the first time that anyone in my group had seen a dead body. To dissect and analyze all the layers and depths was an intellectually and emotionally challenging experience. We had a ceremony at the end of that term to thank all the individuals who donated their bodies to improve medical care for future patients. We learned the names of our cadavers and some of their story about who they were. It was really moving.

Dr. Kosowsky: There are some other important first-year classes. **Physiology,** for example: what does each organ do? How are they related to each other? I was particularly interested in the dynamic aspects of physiology. The human body is such a perfect machine, and it's incredible how it responds to change. One example: when we are exercising, there is demand on our muscles to have more oxygen, so our heart beats faster. We breathe faster and deeper. Our blood vessels dilate so that they can carry more blood.

These are important concepts to avoid misdiagnosis: when patients are having symptoms, doctors always have to ask, what systems that are supposed to be working aren't? Why isn't compensation working as it should? Some systems can compensate up to a point, and then abruptly crash, like a motor revving faster and faster to compensate for a loose gear shaft, until a key component burns out, grinding everything to a halt. Other times, the body's compensatory responses to an injury undermine the healing process or end up being counterproductive in other ways (like during allergic reactions, where the body's own immune system attacks itself). I illustrate these as examples of the complexity of what may be going on when a patient comes in with particular set of symptoms; there is a lot to sort out, and by its very nature, the body's complexity defies cookbook thinking.

The second year of medical school builds upon the basic foundation of how a normal body works to delve into **pathophysiology:** what happens when things go wrong. For each disease, medical students learn about what causes it, how it manifests, and how to diagnose and treat it. They begin to learn the classic presentations of diseases and how to recognize simple patterns. Crushing chest pain in a middle-aged male? Think heart attack. Headache accompanied by flashing lights? Think migraine. This pattern recognition forms the basic framework for teaching students how to make a diagnosis.

Medical students also learn additional key concepts, such as the difference between symptoms, syndromes, and diagnosis. **Symptoms** are the "complaint" that the patient came in with, for example, a cough, shortness of breath, or a headache. **Syndromes** are patterns of symptoms that appear together and are related in some way. Runny nose, fever, and muscle aches brings to mind a viral syndrome, for example. A **diagnosis**, on the other hand, implies an underlying and unifying explanation or cause. Inflammation of the appendix causes appendicitis, which is the diagnosis of a particular disease. These are concepts important to how doctors-in-training learn to process information—and important to keep in mind when the doctor is explaining what you might have.

Concurrently, medical students begin to learn how to take a medical **history** and conduct a **physical exam.** Having never been detectives, we are not sure if the analogy holds, but perhaps learning the history is akin to learning how to interview a witness. Initially, the student is focused on learning the key components of a generic history; later, the student spends time watching how master clinicians use various techniques to elicit the subtleties of the history that vary from patient to patient.[1]

Medical students often carry a template with them so that they don't forget all of the elements of the history. Initially, the template functions as a kind of checklist, that has a specific order:

COMPONENTS OF THE HISTORY	DEFINITION
Chief complaint	The reason why the patient is seeking medical attention
History of present illness	Detailed description of the above
Past medical and surgical history	Prior medical diagnoses and past surgeries
Medications	A list of all medications and dosages that the patient is taking
Drug allergies	Known allergies to medications and nature of adverse reaction
Family history	What diseases run in the family
Social history	Smoking, drinking, and illicit drug history; occupational history; in general, what the patient does when they are not in the hospital
Review of systems	A list of the body systems and the symptoms associated with them

You have already heard about some of these elements, in particular the **chief complaint** (the reason why the patient is seeking medical attention), and the **review of systems** (a list of all the body systems and symptoms associated with them). We present the entire template here in order to show that while it is a useful device for the novice to think of the history in a generic and linear way, trained doctors are meant to get beyond the tool itself; the template should not be used as a questionnaire. The template does provide a framework for thinking through a patient's history, and that's the reason doctors continue to use it well beyond their training. It is also useful as a communication tool with other doctors to share information about the patient so that they are all on the same page. The mistake is to think of the template as a recipe for obtaining the history: the process of listening to the patient's story is more dynamic than any set recipe can capture.

Dr. Kosowsky: I tell my students to take a history by listening to the story, asking how and why questions, and starting to make connections in their minds. I tell them to use the template checklist in two ways: first, if they get stuck and can't remember what to ask about; and second, as a final check at the end, to make sure that all the bases have been covered.

After the medical history comes the physical examination. To continue with the detective analogy, if the medical history is like questioning the witness, the physical exam is like hunting for evidence at the scene of the crime.

✚ 911 ACTION TIP

Most doctors will incorporate some aspect of the template in their history-taking. Beware if your doctor appears unable or unwilling to deviate from a templated history. For example, if you mention an additional symptom, or a new detail like you've stopped taking a medication, your doctor should stop and ask you more about these issues instead of moving on to the next item on the list.

Dr. Wen: I remember the process of learning the physical exam to be a harrowing experience. You have to learn to touch patients and figure things out about the size and health of their organs! Listen to the heart and lungs and make sense of it! Look into ears and eyes and noses and throats and elicit information! While all the time learning to be comfortable about violating people's personal space.

As medical students, we got to practice the physical exam on each other first. There was a session every week where we got into pairs and practiced, say, the abdominal exam on each other, and learned how to feel for the liver and spleen. One of our professors told us about how, when he was in medical school, he found that his physical exam partner's spleen was enlarged—this guy turned out to have lymphoma. Nothing like that happened to me, thank goodness, but getting comfortable with the physical took a lot of getting used to.

Medical students are supposed to learn that the physical exam can't be interpreted in isolation. Each clue is just one of many pieces of the puzzle. Almost every physical finding can be conceived along a spectrum from "normal" to "abnormal." Take height, for example, or shoe size. There is a range that is typical, but at what point does one become "abnormally" short or have an "abnormally" large shoe size? Medicine defines "normal" at the 95th percentile, which automatically means that 5 percent of people who are actually "normal" are, by definition, pegged as abnormal. Trainees eventually learn that "normal" is often not as useful of a clue as symmetry (e.g., if breath sounds are different on two sides of the chest), change (e.g., if there is a new heart murmur or if one has been there all along), or severity (mild tenderness to deep palpation versus severe tenderness with just light touch).

✚ 911 ACTION TIP

Keep these concepts of symmetry, change, and severity in mind when you are talking to your doctor. Many patients find it hard to communicate their symptoms. It helps to talk about how one leg feels different from the other (symmetry), how your shortness of breath has changed from when you're walking to all the time (change), and how your belly pain is keeping you awake at night (severity).

. . .

Just like a detective must learn to collect clues before she analyzes them, the budding physician must first learn to gather information through practicing the history and physical. It's during the "clinical" years of medical school, the third and fourth years, that students rotate through various medical specialties and learn "on the job." It's during this part of their training that medical students begin to figure out how to interpret the seemingly disparate information they garnered from the history and physical.[2]

What they aim to do eventually is to solve the whodunit: what does the patient have—what is the **diagnosis?** A diagnosis identifies the nature and cause of the patient's symptoms, anything from a simple cold to a life-threatening brain aneurysm. For a given diagnosis, the doctor then considers the **natural history** of the disease: how the disease impacts the body, how long the disease is supposed to last, and so forth. (A cold may typically last a few days to a week; a brain aneurysm may be stable for years but may also lead to rupture.)

When applied to the individual, the natural history becomes the **prognosis**—that is, the likely outcome of the disease. That's because the natural history of a particular process often varies by the individual. Pneumonia in a healthy young woman leads to minor inconvenience; pneumonia in an elderly nursing-home resident who has many medical problems may be fatal.

The natural history is also affected by outside influences, including deliberate attempts to modify outcomes—what we know as **treatment.** Will the patient benefit from antibiotics? Surgery? Or is watchful waiting an equally good option? What are the side effects and benefits and risks of each type of treatment? Ultimately, figuring out the treatment and making the patient feel better is the end goal. However, to get there, doctors need to understand the natural history and how it can be modified, and in order to get to that point, it all starts with getting to the right diagnosis.

Initially, medical students learn about diagnosis through simple **pattern recognition**. A few key words or phrases spark the "ah ha!" moment. Eavesdrop on a group of medical students and one will inevitably hear references to everything from classic signs of common diseases ("elephant sitting on chest . . . heart attack!") to some esoteric references ("abdominal pain after a scorpion bite . . . must be pancreatitis!").[3]

Medical students also begin to learn "rules" that are supposed to trigger their recognition of certain diseases. For ease of memorization, signs and symptoms are often grouped together, as in 3s ("triads") or 5s ("pentads"). Jaundice, fever, and right upper quadrant abdominal pain? That's the famous "Charcot's triad" of ascending cholangitis—a serious infection of the bile duct! Anemia, low platelets, kidney failure, confusion, and fever? The classic pentad signifying thrombotic thrombocytopenic purpura—a rare, and very serious, blood disorder!

Sooner or later, when medical students encounter real patients on the wards, they learn that these "rules" only get you so far. That's because real patients don't always have classic signs and symptoms, and, when they do, it takes time to sort out which symptoms are the important ones. Students soon realize why diagnostic acumen is a skill held in such high regard— and why medical mystery shows like *House, M.D.* and the *New York Times* column by Dr. Lisa Sanders[4] are so popular.[5]

Figuring out how to make the diagnoses rests on the concept of the **differential diagnosis.** By now, we know what the differential diagnosis is *not*. We know that it is *not* simply a list of things of worst-case scenarios to be "ruled out." Just because a diagnosis is theoretically possible doesn't mean that every patient needs to have it be considered; in most cases, that would be as arbitrary and unnecessary as thinking that any person walking down the street could be an ax-murderer.

We also know that worst-case reasoning doesn't get the doctor to the actual diagnosis the majority of the time. In certain situations, it may be important to consider the worst-case possibility, but to arrive at an actual diagnosis, you also have to be thinking about the most likely diagnosis.

That's where the differential diagnosis comes in. We define the differential diagnosis as the range of possible diagnoses (including combinations of two or more diagnoses) that might reasonably account for the patient's presentation. A patient comes in with a cough: this brings up a whole host of possibilities, from a cold, to pneumonia, to lung cancer and tuberculosis. Each potential diagnosis can be assigned a likelihood ranging from very high (say greater than 99 percent) to very low (say less than 1 percent). Rarely in medicine (as in anything else) is there 100 percent certainty, meaning that the differential diagnosis is usually populated by several potential diagnoses of varying probabilities. Depending upon how specific or nonspecific the presentation, how certain or uncertain the doctor is about a particular diagnosis, and how thorough the doctor needs to be in terms of considering the more remote possibilities, a differential diagnosis can include any number of diagnoses. If one adds up the likelihoods of all the items on the differential, the sum total of all the likelihoods is close to 100 percent.

We say "close to" 100 percent because the actual percentage can sometimes be a little bit higher or a little bit lower. How can that be? Well, sometimes, patients can have two diagnoses at the same time. For example, a patient has calf pain. The doctor thinks it's probably a muscle strain (the pain started a week ago after playing tennis), but she's also considering the diagnosis of a deep venous thrombosis, a blood clot in the leg, which could potentially be more serious. Let's say these are the only diagnoses she's considering. Simple enough, right? Except that it's also not inconceivable that the patient has *both* a muscle strain *and* a blood clot. "Quite a coincidence that would be!" you'll say. "Is it even worth considering the likelihood of having *two* diagnoses?" Well, perhaps. As it happens, recent trauma is one of the conditions that predispose people to blood clots in their calves. So in this case, because the diagnoses are related, it may not be unreasonable at all to consider the possibility of having both. It wouldn't be such a coincidence.

It's also OK if the numbers add up to a number less than 100 percent. But wouldn't that imply that we're leaving out some possibilities? The answer is yes. Even the most astute clinician can't be expected to list every possibility, down to the rarest, most unusual diagnosis. New syndromes are described in medical journals every day and new diagnostic categories are proposed all the time, implying that there are others out there that have yet to be discovered. Recognizing that some problems defy diagnosis, the medical community has even come up with terms to describe such conditions, like "idiopathic" (arising spontaneously or from an unknown cause), "cryptogenic" (of hidden or mysterious origin), "primary" (without a first cause), and "atypical" (not associated with usual diagnostic categories.)

Acknowledging this, any doctors with common sense and an ounce of humility would be willing leave a percent or two in the "unknown" category when tabulating her differential.

Dr. Kosowsky: The differential diagnosis is one of my favorite topics. I try to come up with a differential diagnosis for every patient I see, and I ask that every student and resident who works with me to do the same. Patients come to doctors because they want us to be thoughtful, and to do this we have to consider a broad range of possibilities. A lot of the time, we'll be fairly certain that we know the diagnosis. The man who has a burning sensation in his chest when he lies down after eating—he probably has heartburn. Depending on the story, I may say that he has a very high likelihood of having heartburn, and deem heartburn to be the most likely diagnosis.

Let's say I'm 95 percent sure that's what it is. But I'm not 100 percent sure. By definition, there must be something else that his symptoms could represent, because something else has to account for the additional 5 percent. To be thorough in my duties as his doctor, I should at least consider what those other things could be. Could it be a heart problem, like inflammation of the lining around his heart? A lung problem like pneumonia? Unlikely . . . but I have to at least think about it. The likelihood of all those other entities may be low, but it's important to think about them and include them in the differential diagnosis.

At a certain point, the likelihood of some of these entities may be so low that these diagnoses can come off the list—if it's just as likely for anyone in the world to have a particular diagnosis as your patient, then it's not part of the differential diagnosis anymore.

Dr. Wen: What we're aiming for in coming up with the differential diagnosis is to make sure that we're being thorough. It's not the same as worst-case scenario thinking, because our emphasis is on getting to the right diagnosis and not just "ruling out" all the bad things. We are also not trying to list every single bizarre disease out there. Remember that our approach to diagnosis is to help you with everyday symptoms and diseases. We're not talking about some one-in-a-million diagnosis that pretty much every astute clinician will miss; we're talking about diseases that you, or your spouse, or your child, could have, that your doctor should pick up. Patients are misdiagnosed all the time, and common things being common, it's the common illnesses that doctors miss.[6]

During their third and fourth years, medical students learn that there are a number of different frameworks for coming up with the differential diagnosis. One framework is to go through by organ system: come up with everything related to the cardiovascular system, the gastrointestinal system, the nervous system, and so on. A related framework is to work anatomically from head to toe to see if it could be something originating from, say, the head or the neck or the chest that somehow causes the symptoms. Yet another is to think through the differential diagnosis is by using the mnemonic VINDICATE:

VINDICATE MNEMONIC	
Vascular	Dealing with the blood vessels and the circulatory system, e.g., clotting disorders, strokes
Infection/Inflammatory	Infections can be bacterial, viral, or fungal; inflammatory diseases involve acting up of the immune system, e.g., allergic reaction
Neoplastic	Having to do with cancer, e.g., new diagnosis of lung cancer
Drugs/Degenerative	Drugs include toxicities from medications as well as illicit substances; degenerative processes occur with aging, e.g., osteoporosis, Alzheimer's disease
Idiopathic/Iatrogenic	Idiopathic means the cause is not known to medical science at this time; iatrogenic is something caused by a medical intervention, e.g., complication of a procedure

(continued)

VINDICATE MNEMONIC	
Congenital	Something a patient is born with, e.g., Down's syndrome
Autoimmune	Autoimmune implies that the body's own immune system is attacking itself, e.g., lupus
Trauma	Occurs as a result of trauma, e.g., hip fracture as a result of fall
Environmental/Endocrine	Environmental is the result of outside influences, e.g., cold or heat exposure; endocrine occurs due to malfunctions in the body's hormones, e.g., diabetes or thyroid disorders

For a particular presentation, the student then works through each of these categories in turn to see if there are any vascular processes, infectious processes, and so forth, that may explain the patient's symptoms.

Yet another possible framework for approaching the differential diagnosis is to consider the timing of symptoms. Certain biologic processes have a characteristic time course, regardless of the organ system at play. An acute process that begins with the sudden onset of symptoms may signal trauma or something involving blood vessels like a hemorrhage or a blood clot. Something that happens over days may be more likely to be infection or inflammation. Symptoms occurring over months may be attributed to a chronic condition like cancer or diabetes.

One can also think of the differential diagnosis in terms of epidemiology, or population likelihoods. A three-year-old has a cough—so one can begin by thinking about what are the most common causes of cough in toddlers. An eighty-year-old has memory problems—one thinks about the most common causes of dementia in the elderly.

Dr. Kosowsky: With all the different frameworks, how does a doctor decide which to use to come up with the differential diagnosis in any particular case? The answer is that it depends—but it often helps to use multiple frameworks at once. I'll give you an analogy: let's say that my wife, Devorah, calls me in the car and asks me to pick up a dozen eggs from the supermarket on my way home from work. Twenty minutes later I'm at the supermarket, and I'm drawing a blank. What was it that I was supposed to buy? I could always call my wife at home, but I don't want to seem like a complete idiot, so I try to figure this out on my own.

There are several ways I can approach this. I can use an "anatomical" framework, walking up and down each and every aisle until I come across the item that jogs my memory. At the same time, I can go through categories in my head: Is it a breakfast item? A lunch item? A dinner item? A snack item? I can also think in terms of "epidemiology": What are common things that run out in the kitchen? Eggs, sugar, milk, and so on. If I'm getting desperate, I can even try an alphabetical approach: Does the item start with an "A"? A "B"? And so on. Most likely, I would use a combination of these approaches.

Dr. Wen: In patient care, just like in Josh's example, doctors often use multiple frameworks, because one framework alone might result in missing something critical. Let's say that Josh is walking through all the grocery aisles. He may not have seen the eggs that his wife wanted because they were by the checkout counter in a special sale, or they happen to be out of stock that day. Similarly, if doctors only go through the organ systems framework, they might miss diseases that aren't clearly associated with a particular organ system because they exert subtle effects on multiple systems. This is why formulating the differential diagnosis is such a critical, yet very difficult, skill to attain.

Dr. Kosowsky: Doctors refer to medicine as a "practice" because clinical skill takes years to learn and a lifetime to perfect. Medical training doesn't finish with medical school or residency; doctors should always aim to improve their skills. Medical societies get this; that's why we require doctors to take continuing medical education courses and pass recertifying exams

---

✚ 911 ACTION TIP

Having a differential diagnosis is critical to your medical care. Your doctor should always be able to give you a differential. If there are only one or two items on the list, learn to ask, "What *else* could this be? Can we think through all the different possibilities for what I could have, please?"

---

to make sure they learn the latest medical advances. But it's not just about learning the latest medical advances: it's also about honing the skills one needs to become a better diagnostician. Cookbook medicine doesn't require practice in this sense; all you have to do is to look at a recipe and apply it to the next patient.

In many ways, the ability to develop a differential diagnosis and the ability to communicate with patients go hand in hand. If a doctor doesn't know what to listen for, he won't hear it. And if he doesn't hear it, he can't make the connections he needs to arrive at the right diagnosis. Patients can help with this. You can become a better storyteller by knowing what to "listen for" in telling your own history—but now we're getting ahead of ourselves![7]

Here's a related concept: the **working diagnosis**. The working diagnosis is the diagnosis (or diagnoses) presumed to be the most likely, at least for the time being. It's the diagnosis upon which a plan of care is initiated, and is also used interchangeably with the term *provisional diagnosis*. Having a working diagnosis allows the doctor to consider and provide a prognosis and natural history before the **definitive diagnosis**—the final, proven diagnosis—is firmly nailed down. The working diagnosis is a prerequisite to figuring out a course of treatment, and is a good start to helping you feel better.

Each time you go to see your doctor, you should walk away with at least a working diagnosis. We say at least because, sometimes, a definitive diagnosis can be made right away. You fell and your wrist hurts. An X-ray shows you have a broken bone in your wrist. That's a definitive diagnosis; you will not need a provisional, working diagnosis because it is 100 percent certain what you have. Many times, though, the diagnosis is not 100 percent clear, but there is a strong suspicion of one or more possible diagnoses. This is the working diagnosis, and you should not leave your doctor without at least knowing what it is.

But can the doctor be sure? you might say. What if tests are not back yet to confirm exactly what diagnosis you have? This is precisely the point. The working diagnosis is not necessarily 100 percent right. There may even be two or three working diagnoses. This uncertainty does not equate to mistreatment or incompetence, but rather thoughtfulness. Having a working diagnosis means that you and your doctor have a pretty good idea of what you have. It's usually enough if you have a plan for how to confirm the diagnosis, how to treat your symptoms in the meantime, and what dangerous things to watch out for. What's not enough is if you just get a list of things that you *don't* have. Rather, your doctor should help you come up with a full differential diagnosis, then narrow it down to the working diagnosis—at every doctor's visit.

In the next several chapters, we will go over how to work with your doctor to think through your history and physical to come up with a differential diagnosis and then a working diagnosis—with you as an equal partner in the process. We want to conclude this chapter with an explanation of how the differential diagnosis and working diagnosis directly relate to the concepts of **probabilities** and **diagnostic testing**.

Each item in the differential diagnosis is like a scientific theory: you start with the hypothesis that a particular diagnosis is causing your symptoms. Evidence then needs to be collected to either support or refute the hypothesis. In some cases, there may be overwhelming evidence to support one diagnosis over the others at the outset. In others, there may be a number of likely diagnoses, and only through further gathering of clues and observations does one diagnosis emerge as the frontrunner.

✚ 911 ACTION TIP

Don't leave your doctor's office without finding out at least what your *working diagnosis is.* If your doctor doesn't respond to this term, other phrases to ask include, "What is this most likely to be?" and "What is the most likely disease that's causing my symptoms?"

Take the case of Leana's husband, Sebastian, who had chest discomfort when his heart was beating very fast. Based on his history alone—his having been diagnosed with a benign rapid heart beat in the past, his description of a "fluttering" in his chest—the probability of the chest discomfort simply being due to the rapid heart beat itself is very high. Let's say it's 80 percent.[8] That means there is a 20 percent chance of some other reason for his chest discomfort: a pulled muscle, pneumonia, blood clots, heart attack—all these can total up to no more than 20 percent.

When his heart stopped beating so quickly and his symptoms went away, that increased the likelihood even more for the rapid heart rate being the cause of the discomfort—say from 80 percent to 90 percent. That means the probability of the other possible diagnoses, both benign and dangerous diseases, now totals 10 percent.

And when the EKGs remains unchanged after two hours, and when laboratory tests are all normal, the likelihood of benign rapid heart rate climbs even higher, to 95 percent, then 99 percent. That means that all the other diagnoses together—including serious things like heart attack and less serious things like heartburn or muscle pull—have less than a 1 percent chance of being true. As more data comes in, that probability continually gets revised.

Presumably, the reason for keeping Sebastian in the hospital and getting more EKGs, blood tests, and a treadmill stress test was to make sure that there wasn't something else wrong with his heart. But what is the likelihood of that? At this point, the chances are already very low. We think it's much lower than this, but let's just say it's one in a thousand, or 0.1 percent.[9] The likelihood of further testing turning up something useful becomes exceedingly low. Yet, this statistic was not presented to Sebastian; instead, he was told that he could die if he didn't stay in the hospital.

Not every decision about diagnostic testing is as straightforward as this. One could see how this would play out differently if Sebastian's presentation was more ambiguous and the likelihood of a heart attack was closer to 10 percent (say if he had never had palpitations before)—neither he nor Dr. Wen would have been so blasé about wanting him to go home! In the real world, there is often a large gray zone when it comes to testing as well, because a lot of times tests need to be ordered, or treatments need to begin, before the doctor is 100 percent sure of the working diagnosis. As more information comes in from the tests, though, the likelihood of various diseases gets modified accordingly. The same thing goes for treatments. In the case of Jerry the mechanic, let's say that ibuprofen completely took away his chest pain. The treatment trial might further confirm that what he had was a muscle pull and not a heart attack.

> It is an old maxim of mine that when you have excluded
> the impossible, whatever remains, however improbable,
> must be the truth.
>
> SIR ARTHUR CONAN DOYLE, *The Adventures of Sherlock Holmes*

The differential diagnosis is a dynamic and challenging concept, one that is critical in figuring out what the patient has. Understanding it, and how probabilities and testing fit into this, will allow for a **diagnostic partnership** with your doctor, and put you on the right track to making sure you are not misdiagnosed.

Congratulations on finishing your crash course in diagnosis! It's time to learn how to work with your doctor to do the detective work required to get to the right diagnosis—without the crutch of cookbook medicine.

911 REVIEW

- It's important to know how doctors learn diagnosis. Patients can use similar methods to help their doctors reach their diagnosis.
- The differential diagnosis is a list of diseases that could possibly account for the patient's symptoms. The working diagnosis is the most likely diagnosis, and is often given provisionally in order to initiate further testing and to begin treatment.
- Every time you see a doctor, you should ask for, and have a discussion about, your differential diagnosis and your working diagnosis.

Eight

Begin at the Beginning

"If you listen carefully, the patient will tell you exactly what's wrong with them." So goes the old medical aphorism. Every patient and every doctor knows instinctively that the patient's story is important. The story is what the patient hopes to convey when they see their doctor, and what the doctor seeks to elicit from the patient. The patient expects the doctor to take the history with precision, sift through the details, and uncover clues to the diagnosis. The doctor engages the patient in conversation, and at the end of the history and physical exam, a diagnosis is made and a treatment plan is decided together.

Unfortunately, this process of carefully probing to arrive at the patient's story is no longer the norm in the practice of modern medicine. In Part II, we demonstrated how the cookbook approach to diagnosis devalues the patient's story. Discrete data from close-ended questions are all that's required; anything more is superfluous and distracting. In this way, cookbook medicine eliminates the need for narrative altogether. In stark contrast is our partnership approach to diagnosis, where the patient narrative—your story about what brings you to the doctor—is the first and most critical component to get to your diagnosis.

In the next two chapters, we will show you how the patient's story serves as the foundation for diagnosis. These chapters lay the groundwork for preventing misdiagnosis. As with previous chapters, the ✚ 911 Action Tips are scattered throughout this section. Part IV contains further Prescriptions for Patients that correspond to these principles.

Getting beyond the chief complaint

> Singularity is almost invariably a clue. The more featureless and commonplace a crime is, the more difficult it is to bring home.
> —SIR ARTHUR CONAN DOYLE, *The Boscombe Valley Mystery*

"Mr. Allen is a twenty-three-year-old man who presents with back pain. . . ."
"Mrs. Davis is an eighty-seven-year-old woman who comes in for difficulty breathing. . . ."

So begins the medical presentation. As we discussed in Chapter 7, first-year medical students learn that the "chief complaint" is the very first part of the medical history they need to nail down, right after the patient's name and demographics. "Back pain," "chest pain," "headache," "nausea"—these are all typical chief complaints, and medical students learn to begin presentations this way so as to encapsulate the *one* problem that the patient is having. Everything after the chief complaint attempts to clarify and expound upon it. Mr. Allen's back pain will be described further: how and when it started, what it feels like, what associated symptoms there may be, and whether it responded to any treatment. Similarly with Mrs. Davis's troubled breathing— the medical student would ask when the breathing problems started, whether it's happened before, and so forth.

This chief complaint becomes central to how the physician thinks about a problem. "Back pain" immediately conjures up a list of possible diagnoses: muscle strain, kidney stone, aneurysm of the aorta, and so forth. Some of these are benign; some are very dangerous. The same with "difficulty breathing." Coming up with a list of diagnoses based on the chief complaint alone is not inherently bad; after all, developing the differential diagnosis has to start somewhere. Beginning a presentation with the chief complaint is something expert clinicians do, too, at conferences and grand rounds, because it focuses their thinking and the attention of the listener. The chief complaint is part of a common grammar used by health professionals to begin relaying a patient's case; indeed, it is the topic sentence of the medical history.[1]

However, the title line of a story should not be confused with the story itself. With Jerry the mechanic, we saw the problems that arise when the chief complaint supersedes the narrative and displaces the rest of the patient's history. Here's another example. Take "epigastric pain"—pain in the upper part of the abdomen. When a fifty-year-old man comes in to the doctor with epigastric pain, the diagnoses that the doctor conjures up relate to organs in that region of the belly: the stomach, the pancreas, the gallbladder, and perhaps a portion of the small or large intestine. Because the upper abdomen is just below the chest, the heart and lungs may also come to mind. Doctors know that other possibilities exist, too, but if one were to rely solely on the chief complaint of epigastric pain, the evaluation would be focused on "ruling out" problems associated with these organs.

Believe it or not, there are algorithms that teach medical students how to proceed based on a single chief complaint. For example, this is how medical students might be taught to approach the patient with a chief complaint of epigastric pain:

Questions to ask in the history:
- When did the pain start?
- Is it always there or does it come and go?
- What kind of pain is it? Sharp, burning, dull . . . ?
- Does the pain radiate anywhere? To your chest? To your back?
- What other types of symptoms do you have with it? Any nausea? Vomiting? Diarrhea? Fever? Chills? Shortness of breath?
- Does anything make it better or worse? Does exercise make it better or worse? What about eating?
- Has this happened to you before?
- Have you treated yourself with anything over-the-counter?

The patient being asked for this kind of history probably assumes he is receiving good care. And perhaps he is, if the diagnosis fits neatly into a clearly defined branch of the "epigastric pain" algorithm. Let's say that the patient has sharp pains in the center of his stomach that's constant and radiates to his back, and is associated with nausea and vomiting. Eating makes it worse. It's happened before and he has been diagnosed with gallstones. By following the checklist of questions, the medical student would accurately diagnose the patient with gallstones pancreatitis. She would be applauded for asking all the right questions and arriving at the correct diagnosis. The patient would be happy and relieved to know his diagnosis, and all would be on track to figure out a plan to manage his problem.

But what if the chief complaint leads you to a dead end, or, worse yet, down the wrong path?

Dr. Kosowsky: Let me tell you a story of what happened on my last shift. I saw that the nurses just brought in a patient who had a chief complaint of "diplopia and dysarthria," something that instantly raised some red flags. Diplopia is seeing double, and combined with dysarthria, or trouble speaking, this could signal a stroke.[2]

One of our best senior residents was already in seeing this patient. A few minutes later, she emerged and told me the following story. The patient, Lynn Rubenstein, was a forty-two-year-old woman who worked as an administrator at a local liberal arts college. Yesterday morning, while standing around the water cooler and chatting with her colleagues, she began to experience the odd sensation of being outside of her body, as if she were watching a movie about herself in real time. She found herself staring straight ahead, trying hard to focus, to the point where her eye were crossing and everything looked double. She heard herself talking, but her own voice sounded distant and slow, "almost like a 45 rpm record being played at 33." She estimated that this might have gone on for about fifteen minutes (although time seemed to slow down, so she couldn't be sure), until at some point several of her colleagues noticed that she seemed "off" and asked if everything was all right. They asked if she wanted a cup of water or to sit down at a nearby desk. By this point, she was beginning to regain her normal sense of self and was embarrassed about having caused a scene.

She was pretty sure that she was OK after the episode passed, but her colleagues were still concerned, and she was having a hard time explaining to herself, let alone to anyone else, about what had transpired. So when her coworkers decided to call an ambulance to take her to the hospital, she went along with it.

Lynn seemed to be acting normally to the paramedics who brought her in to the ER, but she had indeed described a period when she was "seeing double" and "speaking funny"—hence the diplopia and dysarthria. When pressed, perhaps in order to justify all the fuss, she would say that she still didn't feel "quite right," but she certainly seemed perfectly fine when she arrived at the ER: composed, engaging, even chatty.

From the way the resident presented the patient to me, I could tell that she had taken a thorough history, albeit with the usual series of questions: when did it start? (About an hour ago.) Did you have a headache? (No.) Has this ever happened before? (Maybe, I'm not sure.) Was the double vision in one eye or both eyes? (I don't know, I didn't check.) Did you have any weakness? (I'm not sure.) And so on. She dutifully went on to perform a thorough neurological examination and couldn't find anything wrong. Nevertheless, she was appropriately concerned about the patient's symptoms, specifically that they could represent warning signs of a stroke. And not just any sort of stroke, but a "brain-stem stroke," a particularly devastating type of stroke that can leave patients quadriplegic, or, worse yet "locked in," fully conscious but unable to respond in any way, other than perhaps to blink their eyes.[3]

After she presented the case to me, I asked the resident what she intended to do. She wanted to send the patient for an MRI of the brain.

"I'm betting it's going to be normal," I said. "Then what?"

"Well, I guess we'll have to call a neurologist to see the patient," she responded.

"Why? So that they can tell you her MRI is normal, too?"

But this was an excellent resident, and she knew that when facing a challenge, she could always call upon research papers—and algorithms—to back her up.

"Actually," she said. "I suppose it's safe to send the patient home. There's an algorithm that allows us to calculate the patient's risk of stroke, the ABCD2 score. If we use the ABCD2 calculator, her risk of going on to have a stroke in the next thirty days is less than 5 percent!"[4]

Interesting. A moment ago we were concerned that Mrs. Rubenstein could be having warning signs of a deadly stroke; now we were thinking about sending her home? If the warning signs were there, shouldn't we try and figure out what was causing them and to try and prevent a full-blown stroke from occurring? And what about that 5 percent—a patient might be willing to accept a 5 percent risk in some cases, but what about a 5 percent risk of going on to have a frankly horrific stroke like the "locked-in" syndrome?

I told the resident that I would go in the chat with the patient, and then the three of us would come up with a plan together. I walked to Mrs. Rubenstein's room, and as soon as I pulled back the curtains, I was struck by how well she appeared. She was sitting up in her stretcher, thumbing through a *New Yorker* magazine (clearly no diplopia now), and engaged me immediately in conversation.

"Well, here I am!" she exclaimed (and no dysarthria, either).

"What a frightening story!" I offered back. "I'm glad to see you back to normal."

"And you know what?" she replied. "I wasn't even feeling that stressed out at work today."

I let the conversation continue, but she had already spilled the beans. We began talking about the things that stressed her out, her battle with depression, her battle to lose the weight that she had gained back after her third gastric bypass revision, how she knows she needs exercise but she's too busy with the end of the academic year approaching, and how it's hard sometimes to get out of bed in the morning, especially on gray days like today . . . and she was weeping.

The diagnosis became apparent. It was the diagnosis I had suspected all along because I had seen her list of depression and anxiety medications and because the anatomy of her symptoms just didn't add up in any neurologic pattern. Her symptoms of feeling outside her body were psychiatric in nature. In common parlance, she was having a nervous breakdown, not a devastating stroke as the resident had been worried about. We spoke some more, and I reassured her that her symptoms weren't so unusual after all, and that she was going to be fine. Ultimately, she thanked me for the time spent talking together and assured me that she would call her therapist as soon as

---

✚ 911 ACTION TIP

It's often instructive for patients to find out what was written down as their "chief complaint." Ask your doctor what she determined to be your chief complaint. You may be surprised by what they say; this could be an opportunity to correct a misunderstanding.

---

she got home. She was grateful not to have to undergo any further testing and for the doctor's note excusing her from work for the rest of the day. And when I sat down with the resident after our shift and reviewed with her what we had learned from this case, she, too, thanked me for teaching her an important lesson about thinking past the chief complaint.

Sometimes, I ask my students to think about what the term *chief complaint* really means. By the very nature of the phrase, we acknowledge that the patient may have a number of "complaints," and it's our intention to focus on the most significant one, the "chief" complaint. But is that really what the patient's narrative boils down to a series of complaints? And who decides which among them is "chief," and on what basis? Is it just whatever the patient happens to mention first to the doctor? Or worse, is it just what the doctor is most comfortable addressing because there is a ready-made recipe to "work up" that symptom? I also wonder whether the word *complaint* has pejorative implications: a complaint is an expression of grievance or resentment. Starting with the presumption, however subtle, that the patient is a whining victim can't be a good thing.

I've accepted that despite the linguistic imprecision, the term *chief complaint* is here to stay. However, I continue to teach that understanding the narrative—and, from the patient's perspective, being sure to tell your story for why you went to the doctor—is far more important than the "chief complaint" itself.

Dr. Wen: There are so many other reasons why the chief complaint is inherently problematic—we've mentioned some of them before. Take how it gets generated in the first place. Often, it's the triage nurse jotting down what she thinks is the reason for the patient's presentation. It may be the words the patient happened to use, or it may be the nurse's interpretation of their symptoms. In Josh's example, what are the odds Mrs. Rubenstein said, "My chief complaint is diplopia and dysarthria"? Very low, right? It's what the nurse interpreted. Other times, the chief complaint may even be written down by the registration clerk, a secretary with no training in medicine.

Here's another example of a misleading chief complaint. I saw a woman being wheeled in from the waiting room who was labeled with the chief complaint of "right upper quadrant pain," that is, pain in the right upper portion of the abdomen. Mrs. Downey was a very pleasant sixty-two-year-old woman who spoke with a raspy smoker's voice and who loved to laugh. I have to admit: I saw the chief complaint and began to ask the standard questions about her abdominal pain: where it was, how long it lasted, what other symptoms she had it, and so forth.

The classic teaching is that the chief complaint of right upper quadrant pain should prompt a search for gallbladder problems, since that's where the gallbladder is located.

On the surface, Mrs. Downey appeared to be a "typical" person to have gallstones. She was middle-age, female, obese, and she said the sharp pains came and went, as one might expect if the gallbladder was going into spasm, trying to pass a stone. She pointed to an area under her ribs on the right side when I asked where her pain was. And she did have more tenderness when I pressed on her belly in the right upper quadrant. All the teaching I got in cookbook medicine kicked in, and I began thinking of tests to look for gallstones.

The more I talked to her, though, the more I could see that something in her story didn't quite match the picture for a gallbladder problem. She never went to the doctor's office, she said, because "life is too short to spend asking other people to do things for you. The key is, make life happen yourself!" Her symptoms had gone on for months; it had taken a lot for her to come to the ER that day.

She looked particularly anxious when the conversation came around to the subject of her smoking. She tried to hide her anxiety by laughing nervously and saying to me, "Sweetie, I stopped drinking alcohol, I'm supposed to eat healthy, and I'm not having sex. No way I'm giving up smoking!"

She had more to say. I let her talk. Her face dropped.

"For the last couple of months, I've had less energy than I usually do," she told me. At night, she was frequently woken up by coughing fits, and sometimes she would cough up blood, which really worried her. Over the last month or so, she had little appetite and lost about twenty pounds.

"I wasn't going to come to the doctor, you know. I hate the whole thing, doctors and hospitals and stuff. No offense. . . . You know what I mean. But then I got this pain under my ribs and it wasn't going away, and I thought, well, maybe it's time to get this checked out."

Now the story was taking shape. The pain might have been her reason for coming to the hospital, and maybe it was what she mentioned to the registration clerk and the triage nurse, but it was not the whole story. It wasn't even her *real* chief complaint. If I had just continued with the recipe to "work up" her abdominal pain, I would have proceeded down a list of questions focused on her gastrointestinal system: whether she had nausea and vomiting, when was her last bowel movement, etc. She may not have brought up her weight loss, the fatigue, and the coughing up of blood; and if we did get around to these symptoms, I might not have known where to put them in the algorithm.

But now, with this woman with months of symptoms and a long smoking history, we had a different story. Mrs. Downey had put off on coming to the hospital for months until something pushed her over the edge. Over the course of our conversation, she told me that it was lung cancer she was worried about. I was worried, too.

As we feared, her chest X-ray showed a mass in the right lower lobe of the lung that was pressing down on her diaphragm. A follow-up CT scan confirmed that she had cancer. We now had an explanation for her right upper quadrant pain. We told Mrs. Downey that we would treat her pain and arrange for her to see an oncologist.

I learned a lot from this case. The first is to be wary of the chief complaint. Patients usually don't come in saying, "My chief complaint is right upper quadrant pain." Somebody else gave it a name. Second, the chief complaint can often be misleading. In this case, focusing on the chief complaint led me astray. Deep down, Mrs. Downey actually knew what she had. We just needed to give her a chance to tell us her story. We also needed to put aside our own comfort with the cookbook recipe for "right upper quadrant pain," and instead consider the patient's narrative. And the patient, in this case, needed to be assertive and say why it was that she came to see the doctor and what it was that worried her.

So what happened with Mrs. Downey? I'm afraid I don't have a particularly happy end of the story. She underwent evaluation in the hospital that showed she had widely metastatic disease, with cancer in her liver and bones. A few days after I saw her in the ER, she went home. She ended up deciding against aggressive treatment of her cancer and opted for hospice care. At least her pain would be treated. I checked her medical record for months after and she never returned. I'd like to think that she lived the last of her days making life happen, and, dare I say, enjoying her cigarettes.

In the cases of both Lynn Rubenstein and Mrs. Downey, if we as the doctors used a cookbook approach, we wouldn't have come up with the correct diagnosis—at least, not right away. Maybe we would have eventually hit on something after searching down a series of blind pathways. Or maybe we wouldn't have given the patient any diagnosis at all. Yet, recipes and algorithms are what doctors continue to turn to. Textbooks of emergency medicine, review articles, and pocket books alike—start with any "chief complaint" and you will find pages filled with rules and pathways.[5]

Dr. Lisa Sanders, an internist at Yale University and the medical adviser to *House, M.D.*, describes a case that she frequently discusses with medical students and residents to illustrate the dangers of the chief complaint. Her patient, an older gentleman, went to the ER and was immediately sent to the highest acuity section because the triage nurse saw his heart rate was 20. A normal heart rate is somewhere between 60 and 100 beats per minute; 20 is very low. "Bradycardia," or slow heart rate, was written as the chief complaint.

"But that's not my problem; the reason I'm here is that I haven't been able to pee!" the patient kept on insisting. It is well known that pain itself can enhance a nervous system response called vagal tone and result in very decreased heart rate. But even though the patient was telling a coherent

---

+ 911 ACTION TIP

If you have one primary symptom, make sure that it is identified accurately as the chief complaint. If you have multiple symptoms, resist the urge by your doctor to make one of those things your chief complaint. "I don't just have chest pain," you can say. "I also have a headache and numbness in my fingers. How can we make sense of these symptoms, too?" The concept of the chief complaint isn't going away anytime soon, but you can help steer your doctor away from it and focus on the bigger picture.

---

story that completely explained why he was there and why his heart rate was so low, it took the doctors four excruciating hours to get beyond the chief complaint to put a Foley catheter to relieve his bladder—and to correct his heart rate.[6]

"Doctors are trained to think about life-threatening problems," says Dr. Sanders. "So when they see a chief complaint that sounds scary, they don't want to stop and figure out the rest of the story. But if they don't do that, they're going to miss the diagnosis and the cause of that life-threatening issue."

At the end of the day, if doctors let the chief complaint entirely drive their diagnosis, they are likely to miss key elements of the history and get the diagnosis wrong. This is where you, the patient, come in! You play an integral part in helping your doctor see beyond the one thing she (or the nurse, or the clerk) pegged as your chief complaint. The next chapter will further demonstrate the importance of your narrative, and how you can make sure your story is heard.

911 REVIEW

- The chief complaint is an important part of how your doctor processes your symptoms, but how it is determined is often arbitrary and can lead to misunderstanding and misdiagnosis.
- It's important that your chief complaint accurately reflects your symptoms. Correct it if it's wrong; add to it if it's incomplete.
- Help your doctor see that the chief complaint is only the beginning, rather than the sum total, of your story.

Nine

What's the Story?

We have moved beyond the "chief complaint"; now you have the rest of your story to tell. As we have been emphasizing, your story—the reason why you came to the hospital—is an essential element to figuring out your diagnosis. However, there are some more barriers standing in the way of the doctor understanding your story.

Questioning the need for questions

Colonel Ross still wore an expression which showed the poor opinion which he had formed of my companion's ability, but I saw by the inspector's face that his attention had been keenly aroused.

"You consider that to be important?" he [Inspector Gregory] asked.

"Exceedingly so."

"Is there any point to which you would wish to draw my attention?"

"To the curious incident of the dog in the night-time."

"The dog did nothing in the night-time."

"That was the curious incident," remarked Sherlock Holmes.

—Sir Arthur Conan Doyle, "Silver Blaze"
in *Silver Blaze* (1893)

"When did your chest pain start? Where does it hurt? Does it radiate?"
"Do you have shortness of breath? Abdominal pain? Headache?
  Runny nose?"

The cornerstone of cookbook medicine is the yes-or-no question, not unlike a "choose your own adventure book." If yes to question 1, then flip to page two; if no, then flip to page ten. In order to progress through the choices, you have to ask questions, and the answers have to be discrete, dichotomous choices. Occasionally you'll come across a recipe that allows for a limited range of answers you can choose from, or some other variable that can be easily entered into an equation. Open-ended "essay questions" have no place in an algorithm because they don't direct you down one pathway or another.

Interestingly, the only time cookbook medicine allows for something like an open-ended question may be at the very outset of the history, when doctors ask something like, "So, tell me what brings you in today." That's because all algorithms begin with a chief complaint and the doctor needs to hear certain buzzwords (like "chest pain" or "headache") before they can launch into whatever recipe they are going to use. This seemingly open-ended question is really just another close-ended question in the sense that if the doctor doesn't hear one of these buzzwords right away, she will press on with questions until she hears something that can be "worked up." Let's say the patient responds with something like "I just don't feel right, doc." The doctor will generally keep pressing until there is something that sounds familiar. ("Are you telling me you have chest pain? Shortness of breath? Headache?") And we've already seen what happens when the chief complaint is set in stone.

In contrast, the cornerstone of our partnership approach to diagnosis is the narrative. Close-ended questions are limiting and confining. Instead, we emphasize open-ended questions, or better yet, open-ended statements that advance the patient's story exclamations. Rather than asking "what," "when," "where," and "whether or not," we emphasize the "how" and "why."

One of our favorite shows is *Car Talk*, a weekly hour-long show on National Public Radio. Tom and Ray Magliozzi take calls from all over the nation about some trouble with their cars. To be sure, they are expert diagnosticians when it comes to cars, but they don't rely on exhaustive questioning to find out what they need to know. Rather, by engaging in playful banter, they learn a lot about the owner, how he drives and maintains the car, and one or two key details about the problem that lead them to figure out what's wrong with the car. With the vehicle in question parked halfway across the country (not much opportunity for a "physical exam"!), they base their diagnosis almost exclusively upon the caller's narrative. Cookbook recipes have no role in their approach.

This mode of open conversation should come naturally to all of us. Think about running into an old friend on the street. You ask them about how they are doing, how their family is, and why it's been so long since you've seen each other. These are open-ended questions. Once you are engaged in conversation, the question-answer-question-answer format fades away into open-ended dialogue. A patient-doctor conversation should be no different, and you can help guide your doctor to make this happen.

Dr. Kosowsky: I teach a course for Harvard medical students in which they take their first steps out of the classroom and into the clinical world. These medical students have spent the previous eighteen months studying anatomy, physiology, and all the other preclinical subjects we talked about in Chapter 7, but most of them have never interviewed a real patient before. Some time toward the end of the semester, once the students have mastered the basic elements of the medical history and are beginning to feel comfortable interviewing patients, I invite them to participate in an exercise I call "No Questions Asked."

Here's how it works. Each student is assigned a volunteer patient with an unspecified problem. The students can spend as long as they like talking with their patients and taking medical histories. When they're done, they present the case to me. The goal at this point in their training is not to arrive at a diagnosis, but just to present a coherent history with the essential elements that may be relevant to the presenting problem. But there's a catch. The students can't ask their patients any questions. That's right: that's why it's called "No Questions Asked." Actually, I make some exceptions. "How" and "why" questions are acceptable—these are really openers to get patients to tell more of their stories. And, of course, questions that come up in ordinary conversation ("Is that your husband who's here with you?") are permitted. Each student starts out with a hundred points, and I subtract one point for every close-ended question asked.

The first reaction I get from my students is this: "This exercise is impossible! How are we going to figure out the what, when, and where? How are we going to get answers to questions about all the possible associated symptoms?"

At this point, I relate to them a story about running into an old classmate of mine at our twenty-fifth high-school reunion. We traveled in overlapping circles during our high school years, but our paths had diverged and we hadn't been in touch for almost the entire twenty-five years. After chatting for less than ten minutes, I knew everything I wanted to know about his life: his career as an IT consultant, his failed marriage, his mother's health problems, and his abiding interest in collecting baseball cards. But, for all the information I had gleaned from our chat, I didn't recall asking him any yes-or-no questions. It was a conversation, not an interrogation. In fact, had I started with a preset list of questions, it's unlikely I would have emerged with the same knowledge.

Without fail, every year, my students raise their eyebrows skeptically. And yet, every year, these students emerge from this exercise with some of the best patient histories I've ever been presented with. It takes a while to adjust to the new rules. Students are so accustomed to the Q&A approach that they often don't catch themselves until after a question has been blurted out, and there are lots of uncomfortable pauses in the interviews that would otherwise have been filled by another in a series of questions. But soon enough they catch on. Instead of asking "When did the stomach cramps start?" (Response: "I'm not sure. I think Tuesday. No, wait. Maybe it was Monday?" Either way, we would be no closer to a coherent history.), they'll say, "Tell me more about how your stomach cramps started." (Response: "Let me think. Oh yes. We had just gotten back from the camping trip, and we were exhausted. The next day, I woke up with this terrible cramping and it felt like I was going to have diarrhea, and . . ."). Now we're getting somewhere, and we can start putting together the story. Could there have been something the patient was exposed to on the camping trip? Could the diarrhea be a clue?

Over the years, I've had hundreds of students go through this exercise. No one has ever gotten a perfect score; it's *really* hard not to ask questions when you're trying so hard to get answers. In the real world, it would be silly to even try to get to a hundred. But I've found as a rule that the students who are able to ask the fewest questions end up presenting the most coherent and the best histories. In almost all of these cases, we can arrive at the diagnosis based on the history alone.

On the other hand, I've found that the more questions asked, the worse the history. Sure, a doctor may get lucky and come up with the elements of the history that she needs to make the right diagnosis; but if she spends all her time asking questions, she may or may not hit upon what's really important. She certainly wouldn't be able to discern what stands out from the patient's perspective, and she'll risk allowing her own biases and preconceptions to color the history.

Imagine that you are a patient with chest pain and you're asked, "Do you have pain in your back?" You may answer yes, or you may answer no, but what does it mean either way? Back pain is exceedingly common, and if pressed to think about it, a lot of patients may admit they have it. Although the doctor may be thinking that the sudden onset of chest pain radiating to the back could signify a tear in the aorta—a true emergency—you probably don't know this. You'll probably wonder why the doctor is asking about your back, and depending on what you imagine to be the reason, you may think the doctor will take your symptoms more or less seriously depending on how you answer the question.

So what's a better way to get at whether the patient is having back pain? It's simple: *don't* ask the question.

"Huh?" my students say. "How can you get such specific information without asking about it? Shouldn't we be concerned about 'ruling out' a problem with the aorta?"

"Tell the patient what you're thinking," I instruct them. "If you're on the right track, the patient will let you know."

Instead of asking about back pain, I would simply offer an observation to the patient: "When I see a patient with the type of chest pain that you're describing, one of my first priorities is to find out if they could be having a heart attack. But I also worry about other rare but serious conditions. One example would be something we call 'aortic dissection,' or a tear in the large blood vessel that delivers blood from your heart to the rest of your body. Patients with certain types of aortic dissection may describe their chest pain as radiating or traveling to the back."

Then I pause and wait to see their reaction. Nine times out of ten, the patient will appear a bit puzzled or will be shaking their head dismissively, or will even say, "Not to worry, I don't have pain like that" or "I may have had some back pain, but I'm certain that it's just the same old pain I have when I sit in a car for too long, nothing like what you're concerned about." And so, even without asking a single question, I have the information I need to move on.

My students often struggle to apply this concept to their history-taking, but residents and attendings later in their career have an even more difficult time avoiding the close-ended questions. That's because it's become so ingrained to ask a standard set of questions that it takes tremendous effort and a major leap of faith to try a different approach. It's so much a part of their medical training that their minds are wired toward thinking of everything as a giant algorithm that needs to be teased out by yes/no, whether/not ques-

---

✚ 911 ACTION TIP

You can help guide your doctor away from close-ended questions. One way is to stop him and ask him what he hopes the question will help answer. "What is the significance if I have back pain?" you can ask. The explanation can help inform you, and also be a good segue for you to tell the rest of your story.

✚ 911 ACTION TIP

If you are faced with a yes-or-no question, feel free to elaborate. If you are asked, "Do you have chest pain?" you can explain that you felt a pull in your chest after you moved some heavy furniture. This type of explanation helps to curb cookbook thinking and further yes-or-no questioning. Your doctor may be schooled in asking close-ended questions, but you can turn them around and answer as if you were asked open-ended ones.

tions. As a result, it's also how patients expect to be treated when they go to their doctor. But this is not right—there is a better way!

Dr. Wen: We physicians want answers, and it's satisfying to have a definitive yes-or-no answer. The problem is that if we just focus on getting an answer, any answer, we may end up getting a wrong answer. Josh likes to call it "garbage in, garbage out": if the question is asked just to be asked, what is the answer good for, except more meaningless data points?[1]

One case I had where I probably wouldn't have figured out the right diagnosis if I had been focused on the yes-or-no questions involved Jessica Tomlinson, an eighteen-year-old basketball player. Jessica was diagnosed with asthma when she was a toddler. Her asthma had been generally well controlled without medications, and she rarely experienced flare-ups of her symptoms. She'd never been hospitalized for the asthma before, and it never limited her physical activity. In fact, she had just received a basketball scholarship to a NCAA Division I university, where she was slated to be the starting point guard.

Jessica's parents brought her to the hospital because she was having an asthma attack and was having more trouble breathing. By the time I saw Jessica, she'd already been seen by a medical student and a nurse. The story they gave me seemed pretty straightforward: history of asthma, asthma attack earlier this month, prescribed albuterol by her doctor, now back with shortness of breath. This was a pretty typical story for asthma.

When I walked into her room, Jessica didn't appear to be in any acute distress, but she and her parents seemed concerned.

"Had you taken your albuterol today?" I asked (then quickly berated myself for asking a yes-or-no question).

"No," she answered.

But why not? Had I gone down the path of asking Jessica and her parents the same close-ended questions—when did it start, did you have fevers, did you have wheezing—I would have gotten some confirmatory answers, but wouldn't have been any closer to the real diagnosis. It turned out that there was much more backstory: over the last month, Jessica had been experiencing "attacks" with increasing frequency. The albuterol inhaler that she kept in the medicine cabinet at home expired years ago, so she went to see her pediatrician, who gave her a new prescription. She tried using the inhaler before practice or during breaks in action, but it wasn't helping.

Two nights earlier, her breathing was particularly bad, so her parents took her to an ER, where they found that her heart rate was high. The doctors told her to cut down on the albuterol because it was increasing her pulse too much. They gave her steroids instead, which also didn't seem to help. That day, her asthma attack was back, and since her parents weren't sure whether to give her more albuterol, they brought her to the ER.

I tried to channel Josh and thought to myself, What would Dr. Kosowsky do at this point? Josh always likes to focus on the social context and how the symptoms affect daily life, because it's through talking about everyday life that more clues are obtained and patterns emerge. This girl was a basketball player, and a really serious one at that, so I started there.

"It must be tough on you to be dealing with all this in the middle of basketball season," I said.

Jessica nodded. It was interfering with basketball quite a lot. She'd be in the middle of practice or worse, in the middle of a game, and all of a sudden, she would feel the shortness of breath coming on, then she would feel really tired and have to stop playing.

"It's, like, totally out of the blue," she said, wringing her hands. "I can't predict it. It's getting to the point I'm afraid to pick up a basketball and shoot around on my own."

"Really?" I asked her. "You have no way of knowing an attack is about to happen?"

"Actually, the first thing I notice is that my heart is beating super fast, like

---

✚ 911 ACTION TIP

When telling your doctor your story, it helps to put your symptoms in the context of your life. What were you doing when the symptoms started? How has it affected your daily life? Has it prevented you from doing anything you usually do?

it's pounding in my chest and sometimes skipping beats. Then I feel winded and faint, and I have to stop playing. The albuterol only makes it worse."

This was beginning to sound less and less like asthma: the unpredictable onset, the palpitations, and the paradoxical response to her albuterol inhaler. When I asked her to think back to her asthma attacks when she was a child, she recalled that they weren't like this at all.

And there it was. Without asking any questions, I now had a new sense of what the diagnosis might be. I obtained an electrocardiogram, which confirmed my suspicion: instead of having the normal sharp spikes we're accustomed to seeing on a typical EKG tracing, she had a shallow up-slope leading into each spike. This is known as a "delta wave," the classic sign of Wolff-Parkinson-White syndrome (WPW), a problem with the electrical conduction within the heart. Instead of the electrical impulses being conducted the normal way from the atria to the ventricles, in Jessica, impulses traveled through a different, abnormal pathway.

Patients born with these "accessory pathways" are often not diagnosed until their teens or twenties when they present with rapid heartbeats. Aside from being a nuisance for the patient who may experience a range of symptoms from shortness of breath to feeling faint and fatigued, WPW can also be associated with life-threatening disorders of the heart rhythm and therefore needs to be diagnosed and treated promptly. In a patient like Jessica, an athlete who was having symptoms during exercise, this was a potentially very serious, even fatal, condition.

The good news about Wolff-Parkinson-White is that there is a cure: cardiologists can snake a wire into the heart and burn away the abnormal conduction pathway. Jessica's story has a happy ending: she was seen by cardiologists that day and successfully underwent the ablation procedure a week later. She was able to go back to basketball and is now a star player for her university.

Getting the story by *not* asking questions is hardly a new concept. An age-old trick used by detectives, lawyers, and reporters alike is to engage the subject in conversation. Before the subject knows it, the story will be there.[2] Bob Edwards, the Peabody–award-winning broadcaster, was a master of this technique when he used to host National Public Radio's *Morning Edition*. He was superb in his use of open-ended statements and pregnant pauses to entice his guest into revealing exactly what it was that he and his listeners were dying to find out. A politician on the hot seat, a reclusive author, a corporate spokesperson—none were immune. No matter what "talking points" they entered with, they all inevitably fell under the spell of Edwards's disarming manner of repeating back a phrase he had just heard, expressing a simple term of surprise or interest, or posing a statement of his own—often just a word or two—as if it were a question, and then just waiting for the guest to take off and run with it. Reporters aim to find out their subject's story without leading questions. Your doctor should, too. And if they don't, you can help them![3]

Becoming a better storyteller

Holmes is a little too scientific for my tastes—it approaches cold-bloodedness. I could imagine his giving a friend a little pinch of the latest vegetable alkaloid, not out of malevolence, you understand, but simply out of a spirit of inquiry in order to have an accurate idea of the effects. To do him justice, I think that he would take it himself with the same readiness. He appears to have a passion for definite and exact knowledge. —SIR ARTHUR CONAN DOYLE, *A Study in Scarlet*

"Mrs. X had some vague chest pain, but she's a poor historian."
"Oh, Mr. Y? He always comes in complaining of everything under the
    sun. I can't make heads or tails of it."

Dr. Kosowsky: We've talked about how some doctors and nurses label patients as "poor historians," meaning they can't give much of their history or that they have a tendency to ramble and not make much sense—like May Gillespie, the activist who fainted at her gym. This seems to me a bit of a cop-out. A good clinician should always find a way to figure out the patient's story.

Dr. Wen: You always tell your residents that there's no such thing as a poor history, only a poor history-taker. Maybe that's being harsh, but I agree that the label of "poor historian" is overused and then ends up being stuck with the patient. Some patients actually begin to think of themselves that way, no doubt after they've had several doctors and nurses cut them off while they're trying to tell their story.

One patient I saw last week, a lovely lady in her seventies who always dressed in her church clothes to go to the doctor, stopped me before I could ask her what brought her in to the ER.

"Talk to my nephew," she said as she handed me her cell phone. "My doctors say I'm no good at explaining anything."

I gave her the phone back, and with a bit of coaxing, she turned out to tell me her story just fine.

Dr. Kosowsky: Sometimes, I see doctors give up on a patient's story because the patient has dementia, or a hearing impediment, or some other infirmity that may impede the history-taking. That's not right. Almost always, if the patient has a story to tell, there's some way to get at it. Even if the patient can't talk at all, *somebody* knows the patient's story. A family member, a home health aide, a coworker—they will have something to say. Eventually, the story will come together, although it may take some time and diligence to put together the pieces.

Dr. Wen: In the face of a difficult story, good journalists wouldn't give up and say, it's too complicated, this one person I interviewed won't talk, or doesn't speak English. They find multiple sources, use multiple methods in their interviews, and then compare notes. The same with detectives. They don't just give up and leave the murder mystery unsolved.

Dr. Kosowsky: Related to the unfortunate term *poor historian* is the notion of the "positive review of systems": that no matter what question you ask the patient, they'll answer in the affirmative and claim that they have the symptom. Remember how with Mrs. Gillespie, it seemed that no matter what she was asked, she would answer yes? Headache? Yes. Chest pain? Uh-huh. Fever, chills, sweats? Yup. The implication is that the patient is some kind of hypochondriac who either has everything wrong with them or nothing at all.

Dr. Wen: I've noticed that when patients report multiple symptoms, doctors either try to connect them in very simplistic ways (such as chest pain + shortness of breath = clot in lungs) or they implicitly question whether the patient is really having these symptoms in the first place. But seemingly disparate symptoms are often connected in complicated, but important, ways. Remember the patient we saw a few months ago, Mrs. Gonzalez?

Dr. Kosowsky: Of course. The first line of the triage note said, "multiple complaints." And do you remember how frustrated everyone seemed that the patient couldn't identify one chief complaint?

Dr. Wen: Right. Her nurse is originally from the Dominican Republic, like the patient. When she told us about her, she was rolling her eyes.

"There you go, another middle-aged Latina with 'total body dolor,'" the nurse said. "Everything hurts.'"

And it was kind of true. Mrs. Gonzalez—or Yolanda as she insisted we call her—was writhing in bed, saying that she hurt all over. It did seem like she had every symptom under the sun. Yes, she had pain in every joint, in every muscle. Yes, she couldn't breathe, she had chest pain, she had a headache, she felt hot and she felt cold. The nurse thought it was funny that she answered yes to having a rash even though there was no sign of a rash on her body.

Dr. Kosowsky: On the surface, Yolanda was a "poor historian" with a "positive review of systems." Part of the challenge was that we were communicating through a professional translator who was accustomed to the standard approach of asking and answering close-ended questions. Yolanda did understand some English, and when we tried to summarize her history, she said something that really stuck with me.

Dr. Wen: It was amazing! She sat up, looked us straight in the eyes, and said in English, "That's not what happened. I tell you what happened." She then proceeded to ask the interpreter to translate, line by line, the order of how her symptoms developed.

✚ 911 ACTION TIP

Your doctor should provide you time and space to tell your story, but if she doesn't, you can help create it yourself. For example, if you encounter an impatient doctor who keeps interrupting you as you're telling the story, it may be helpful to tactfully point out, "Doctor, I am trying to explain to you what is going on. I need you to listen to the whole story." Framing it in terms of *your* needing to explain fully will help cushion the message for him.

Dr. Kosowsky: What came out was a story that revealed a lot about her— and led us to her diagnosis. It went something like this. Yolanda's twin granddaughters were born last year, and she arrived from the Dominican Republic three months ago to meet them for the first time. Last month, her daughter and son-in-law took time off from work so they could do a bit of touring and sightseeing together. A few days after returning from a weekend trip to Cape Cod, Yolanda noticed a rash on the side of her neck that seemed to be getting bigger. It was faintly red and didn't itch at all, and after a week or so it disappeared. Then she started having joint pains and feeling more fatigued. These symptoms she attributed to "arthritis" and the fact that she was away from the comfort of her own home. But a few days after that, she began to have pains in her chest and a hard time catching her breath, especially while lying down. Her daughter found her having to sleep on four pillows and convinced her to come in to the ER.

Dr. Wen: By the way, I think it's ironic that the nurse had written down "no" to recent travel. Supposedly Yolanda answered "yes" to everything, and the one time she said "no," it turns out not even to be accurate!

Dr. Kosowsky: That's exactly the point. Close-ended questions like that have limited value when all you're doing is collecting information without really knowing what you're looking for.

Dr. Wen: Right. Once we heard the story, we immediately suspected that what Yolanda had was Lyme disease. Lyme disease is an infection spread by the deer tick. Each symptom separately made no sense, but together, the rash, the joint aches, the fatigue, and the travel to Cape Cod, made us point to the diagnosis of Lyme.

Dr. Kosowsky: One of the complications of Lyme disease is inflammation of the lining of the heart, a condition known as pericarditis. The most common symptom of pericarditis is chest pain of a character exactly as Yolanda described. In the ER, we obtained an ultrasound of her heart, which showed fluid in the lining around Yolanda's heart. We admitted her to the hospital for treatment with antibiotics and anti inflammatory medication. Two days later, her blood work came back confirming the diagnosis of Lyme disease.

Dr. Wen: "If you listen carefully, the patient will tell you exactly what's wrong with them." That was one of the first things you taught me. This is a case in point. If we had simply designated one of Yolanda's symptoms to be the chief complaint and followed an algorithm for "fevers" or a pathway for "joint aches" or "chest pain," we may not have come up with anything. Yolanda would have been labeled another "poor historian" with "multiple complaints." We would have missed an important diagnosis.

In this case, it was the patient who understood that we were getting it all wrong and got us back on track. She was the one who said, whoa, you're not listening to me. Let's start over. You may not be piecing together everything yet, and I may not know what these symptoms mean, but let's work together

---

✚ 911 ACTION TIP

Learn from Yolanda. *If you are concerned that your story isn't being heard, stop and ask your doctor about her understanding of your story.* Ask her to summarize what she knows of your story so far. If it isn't right, start your story over. Your story is the key to your diagnosis, and you should make sure it's heard and understood.

+ 911 ACTION TIP

If you speak another language and do not feel that you are able to communicate all your thoughts in English, try to get a family member or friend who is fluent to accompany you. Make sure they understand your story. If nobody is able to come with you, ask for a professional translator. Meanings can still be lost in translation, so be attuned to the responses of the healthcare provider. If their responses seem incongruent with what you would expect, clarify with the translator. Communication is difficult enough when it is two people involved who do speak the same language; if there is more than one language and more individuals involved, you should do what you can to optimize your chances of getting the story right.

---

and give this a shot. Few patients actually do this, but her approach was incredibly powerful.

Dr. Kosowsky: The story doesn't always turn out to be as dramatic or as ultimately satisfying as in this case. There are many conditions that are associated with "multiple complaints": chronic diseases, depression, substance abuse, domestic violence, even the aging process itself. There may not be a classic presentation of a disease or definitive diagnostic test, and—sadly—there may be no effective cure. Still it's the doctor's job to piece the story together, separate the wheat from the chafe, and arrive at a reasonable differential diagnosis (and then the working diagnosis). Needless to say, without the patient's active participation in this process, it's next to impossible.

Dr. Wen: We doctors need to be a lot better about listening to our patients' stories. What Yolanda illustrated is that our patients can help us by making sure their story is heard. Storytelling is a skill, something that doctors and patients should both work to improve.

911 REVIEW

- Close-ended, yes-or-no questions add little value to the doctors' understanding of your illness.
- Far more important is making sure your doctor listens to and understands your story.
- You can help your doctor be a better listener by becoming a better storyteller.

Ten

What Does the Story Mean?

You've told the doctor your story. Now what? Most of the time, the doctor scribbles a few notes, gets up, and continues on. Depending on why you went to the doctor's office or the ER, you might have your throat checked, your heart and lungs listened to, or your abdomen pressed. Maybe at some point after the doctor leaves the room, you have your blood drawn, or you are sent for an X-ray or some other test.

Something must have been going through the doctor's head as he heard your story. At some point, the doctor must have thought about your differential diagnosis, maybe even came up with a working diagnosis. Yet, more likely than not, you were left out of the loop during these critical decision points that lead from the story to the diagnosis. No wonder your doctor didn't get it right!

To help your doctor do better, you need to become a partner in your own diagnosis each step of the way. It's not just partnership for its own sake; there are real consequences when the patient is not integrally involved in the decision-making process. In this chapter, we discuss how patients can take an active role in the diagnostic process, from the history to the physical exam to the differential diagnosis.

Sharing in the thought process

> "Poirot," I said. "I have been thinking."
> "An admirable exercise my friend. Continue it."
> —AGATHA CHRISTIE, *Peril at End House*

Dr. Wen: The consumer empowerment movement has been very effective in getting patients involved in the decision-making process when there is a treatment to be selected. Should you start this cholesterol-lowering medication or try to control your cholesterol with diet? Should you begin treatment for your cancer with chemotherapy or with surgery and radiation? There are all kinds of tools to help you make these treatment decisions. One area we need to get better at is to empowering patients to participate in what may be even more important: the diagnostic process.

Getting involved in how your diagnosis is made starts at the very beginning. As you're telling your story, ask what your doctor is thinking. It will give you an opportunity to correct any misconceptions, add additional history, and even refute some theories. I've had patients with abdominal pain tell me they've had "no surgeries," but when I express concern about appendicitis or gallstones, they tell me not to worry about that, because they've already had their appendix and gallbladder removed. That certainly helps to narrow my differential diagnosis!

Dr. Kosowsky: It's frequently cited that up to 90 percent of diagnoses can be made by history alone. It's possible that the number is even higher than that. With the availability of modern technology and abundant recipes, today's doctors often take shortcuts with their histories and turn to testing as a substitute. What they're not seeing is that no test has ever been shown to be as effective as the history—not even close.

We live in amazing times. There are tests that doctors can use to tailor therapy for cancer and other diseases based on the patient's individual genetic information. This is what's known as "personalized medicine" or "genomic medicine"; these movements are incredibly popular and attract millions of dollars of research funding. However, when it comes to diagnosis, doctors don't generally need to delve into an individual's DNA; something that is virtually free—the history—usually holds the answer! We advocate for a type of personalized medicine that involves taking a personalized history, performing a personalized physical exam, and approaching each patient as an individual rather than as a list of variables to be plugged into an algorithm. The patient is really the only one who can try to get their doctor to do that.

Sound cheeky? Before you dismiss this as too far out of your comfort zone, here's another reason to ask your doctor for her thought process: asking your doctor early on about what she makes of your story is an excellent way to curb cookbook thinking. Say you came into the ER with bronchitis, but because you reported discomfort while coughing, you were labeled with a chief complaint of chest pain. Your doctor sees "chest pain" and is worried you could have had a heart attack. She asks you a bunch of questions, then wants to keep you for tests of your heart. This is the chance to ask her: do you think my heart attack would cause my hacking cough or my fever? Pretty soon, you are back on track. Having this discussion will help lead your doctor away from the cookbook mind-set and focus her back on your particular presentation and your personalized history. Asking about and understanding your doctor's thought process leads to better care for you, so why not do it?

✚ 911 ACTION TIP

As you are telling your story, ask what the doctor is thinking. "What are you thinking so far could be the cause of my symptoms?" If he says he can't be sure yet, reassure him. "Of course, but I'd like to understand your thought process. What are the things you are thinking based on what I've said to you?" Sharing in the thought process is a critical part of being an equal partner in your care.

Participating in your own physical exam

It seemed to me that a careful examination of the room and the
lawn might possibly reveal some traces of this mysterious individual.
You know my methods, Watson. There was not one of them which
I did not apply to the inquiry. And it ended by my discovering traces,
but very different ones from those which I had expected.

—Sir Arthur Conan Doyle, *The Crooked Man*

In Chapter 2, we discussed how the Era of Depersonalized Diagnosis has
deemphasized and devalued the laying on of the hands during the physical
exam. Recently, a movement started at Stanford Medical School to "bring
back the physical exam."[1] "The Stanford 25," as it is called, consists of a set of
twenty-five diagnostic maneuvers and clinical signs that the group believes
should be learned and practiced by medical students. Their point is that in
this modern era where we rely so much on blood tests and advanced imaging for diagnosis, doctors are neglecting a critical diagnostic test (second
only to the history): examination of the patient.

"Hold on here," you might be asking. "My doctor does examine me!
Every time I see a doctor, there's a physical exam."

Certainly, every medical encounter includes a physical exam, but for
many doctors, the physical has become a part of the ritual, a checklist of
things that must be done without a clear indication for what is being sought
(yet another reason to have the conversation with your doctor early about
what they are looking for on the exam). Ask yourself this: how often did
your doctor explain to you what was a normal or abnormal physical finding?
How often did your doctor tell you what your physical exam implied about
your diagnosis?

Dr. Wen: I had a patient, Dr. Al Montrose, an eighty-two-year-old retired
dental surgeon who came in with what sounded like a respiratory infection:
he had a few days of congestion and sneezing, and then developed a high
fever and shaking chills. He wasn't coughing much, and his lungs sounded
pretty clear—but his symptoms seemed to suggest a diagnosis of pneumonia.

A few hours into his ER visit, after his chest X-ray came back normal and labwork revealed nothing, his blood pressure began to drop. It wasn't until then that I did a complete head-to-toe exam, and found that he actually had a raging skin infection in his left foot. Because of his diabetes, he hadn't felt much pain, but the infection had spread from a small area of skin breakdown in his great toe to involve almost the entire foot. We started IV antibiotics right then—but a few hours later than we should have.

Dr. Montrose turned out OK, and his foot was salvaged, but I'll always remember that lesson. I should have discussed with him earlier about how his story didn't quite fit the diagnosis of pneumonia and asked for his help in what to look for on the physical exam. For example, other things that could have caused shaking chills would include flu (perhaps, but he had been vaccinated), urinary tract infection (always possible in the elderly, but he had no symptoms), abdominal infection (unlikely, if he did not complain of any pain and was not tender on exam), and skin or soft tissue infection (usually associated with pain, but in a diabetic patient, not necessarily—so it would be important to undress him and examine fully). Had I gone through this process with him, we would have decided together to look elsewhere for a source of infection. He might have offered that he had noticed some redness in his big toe, and I would have found it. Instead, I almost missed a life-threatening condition.

Another case that was just as instructive involved Mrs. Nancy Kellogg, a forty-five-year-old biotech executive who came in with a swollen and tender right lower leg. She thought the swelling developed over the course of a few days. The pain had become unbearable, particularly when she was walking.

The other thing that came out in her history was that everyone in her family had a blood-clotting disorder. Her leg was swollen and painful, and with her family history, we had to make sure it wasn't a blood clot. That was the most life-threatening disease; surely we needed to "rule out" that bad diagnosis?

We ordered an ultrasound of her leg veins, but there was no clot. We ordered an X-ray, but there were no fractures. Her leg wasn't red and she didn't have a fever; this was not an infection, either.

What was going on? I had no clue. An astute attending physician happened to be passing by and I asked him to take a look at Mrs. Kellogg. He carefully examined her leg, palpating top to bottom, asking her where it hurt most. It didn't take long for him to figure this out.

"It's a medial tibial plateau fracture," he told me.

What about the X-ray? It said there were no fractures! We went back to look at it with the radiologist. As it turned out, a second look at the X-ray found that there was a hairline fracture in her leg, right where the pain and tenderness was centered—and right where the other doctor said it was. The physical exam finding was missed because we weren't looking for it—we'd been focused entirely on "ruling out" the blood clot. And because it was so subtle of a finding, the radiologist wasn't looking for it and missed it, too. All of us had focused on a small piece of the puzzle—a piece that, as it turned out, turned out to be irrelevant—and neglected to focus on the part of the physical exam that was most important.

When I went back to my patient with this diagnosis, she lit up. "Yeah, I knew that's where it hurt the most!"

Indeed, she did. Had we involved her more in the physical exam, it would have become clear that her pain could be localized to an area that would didn't correlate with a blood clot, but rather with a fracture.

Dr. Kosowsky: Your stories remind me of a lady I saw with a missed diagnosis. Actually, this is not just a case of one miss, but fifteen. Eileen Mc-Cullough is a twenty-four-year-old rather obese young lady who had undergone an appendectomy a year before. In the last five months, she'd been plagued with bouts of severe abdominal pain. At times, the pain that was so bad that she had to go to the ER—fourteen times, in fact. The time I saw her was number fifteen: that's right, the fifteenth visit to the ER in five months.

During these past fourteen visits, Eileen had been seen by some of my excellent colleagues, emergency physicians and surgeons, attendings and residents. Everyone had been appropriately concerned about her pain: in someone with this much pain after an operation, it could signify an infection, an obstruction, or some other complication of her surgery. As a result, Eileen had received no less than eight abdominal CT scans and five ultrasounds. Every test, so far, had been "negative," and every time, she had been sent home just to return with recurring bad abdominal pain.

Well, I wanted to see if I could solve this problem for her once and for all. My resident that day wasn't so optimistic.

"She's already been here fourteen times," he complained. "How can we make any difference to her this time? I don't think we can avoid doing a CT, but what are we going to find that's any different?"

"Probably nothing, not with another CT," I said. "But how about we start from the beginning? Let's find out more about this pain that she has."

"But people have already done the 'workup,' " he said. "Why are we reinventing the wheel?"

"Because they haven't gotten it right," I responded. "If they had, she wouldn't have come back. We're going to get it right this time."

As skeptical as the resident was that lucky number 15 would be any different, he set off on the mission. Before long, he came back with an excited grin on his face. It turns out that Eileen's pain was a colicky, crampy pain. It was often not there, but when it was, it was severe. It was worse when she bent over or changed positions. She felt fine otherwise. She just wanted to know what was causing this pain. She pointed to one exact location on her abdomen, just to the right of her belly button, as the point where her pain emanated.

"And you know what happened when I pressed on that spot?" the resident said, excited. "I felt a hernia!"

In a matter of minutes, this resident had solved what dozens of top-rate doctors and tens of thousands of dollars of imaging tests could not. He didn't just ask her a list of questions—he listened to what she had to say. He didn't just do a cursory exam—he did a focused physical exam that fully involved the patient.

✚ 911 ACTION TIP

Be involved in your physical exam. Point out exactly where your pain is. Demonstrate what makes your pain better or worse. Ask your doctor what she is looking for. Inquire about any abnormal findings. You should feel perfectly comfortably saying, "I just want to make sure I understand what's going on with my body."

He was right. When we looked back at the CT scans, we could actually see the tiny hernia. It was so small that the radiologists hadn't picked up on it before, but since we knew exactly where on the belly it was, they were able to find it on the scan. Yet another reason to know what you're looking for before doing a test, rather than to use the test as the end-all-be-all of diagnosis!

The resident had done a great job, and I was proud of him. Of all of us, though, it was Eileen who was the happiest to know of her diagnosis at last.

"The pain is bad, but it's not knowing what it could be that was the worst part," she told us. "Now that I know what it is, I can live with the pain."

Or without it. Eileen has since gotten surgery to fix the hernia, and we haven't seen her back in the ER for any more pain.

911 REVIEW

- Personalized medicine also entails a personalized approach to making your diagnosis.
- Ask to share in your doctor's thought process from the beginning. Even before he conducts a physical exam, ask him what he thinks is going on—what he has so far as your differential diagnosis.
- Participate in your physical exam. Point out what worries you, and ask your doctor what she is finding as she examines you.

Eleven

Help Me Help You

If you have to go to a doctor, you probably wouldn't voluntarily choose someone who practices cookbook medicine. The bad news is that as a result of their training and the pressures of the healthcare system, many doctors practice this way. The good news is that you—the patient—can change the way your doctor practices medicine. In each individual encounter, you can make sure that your doctor is giving the best care possible for you. Every encounter with you and with people like you will add to the doctor's appreciation that there is a better way to diagnose patients. This approach, shared by you to your doctor, will help that doctor become a better doctor for you and avoid misdiagnosing you. It will help them become a better doctor for their other patients and a better teacher to future doctors.

In this chapter, we demonstrate how you can continue the partnership with your doctor and make sure you receive excellent, individualized medical care. Everything goes back to the diagnosis, so let's talk about what happens once your history and physical exam are complete.

Making a differential diagnosis together

As Cuvier could correctly describe the whole animal by the contemplation of a single bone, so the observer who has

thoroughly understood one link in a series of incidents should be
able to accurately state all the other ones, both before and after.
—Sir Arthur Conan Doyle, *The Five Orange Pips*

Recall that in order to make a diagnosis, doctors have to start out with a
differential diagnosis: a list of possible diseases to account for the patient's
symptoms and their relative likelihoods. Coming up with a list of differential diagnoses requires that the doctor consider the most likely diagnoses as
well as rarer conditions that may be important not to miss.

Is a differential diagnosis always necessary? Absolutely! As we explained
in Chapter 7, the differential diagnosis is all about probability, so if it's not
100 percent certain that someone has one disease, there must be a probability of other diagnoses. Almost never is the diagnosis 100 percent clear, so it
behooves the doctor—and the patient—to consider other possibilities.

Before we talk about how to come up with the diagnosis, let's review the
four categories of differential diagnoses:

#1. Good stories for common conditions. A differential diagnosis
for this category is the easiest to come up with. Common things being
common, they are the most easily recognized by the doctor and patient alike, and are often at the top of the list. A ten-year-old boy, who,
along with half his classmates, has been home with vomiting and diarrhea, likely has viral gastroenteritis—the common "stomach flu." A
thirty-year-old investment banker with stomach aches after loading
up on ibuprofen probably has gastritis.

This is classic pattern recognition. Medical students are taught
early on to think about the common conditions first, especially if the
story is a typical one. "When you hear hooves, think horses, not zebras," the saying goes. It's important to consider the less common
things as well, but thinking about classic presentations of common
conditions can get you well on your way toward a working diagnosis.[1]

#2. Not-so-good stories for common conditions. A migraine headache is a common condition in young people. Classically, patients experience throbbing headaches along with nausea, vomiting, and light

sensitivity. Some patients experience an "aura" of visual symptoms, with sparkling lights in their peripheral vision before the headache starts. Less commonly, this "aura" may involve numbness, tingling, and other sensory symptoms. This is a less typical presentation, but for a twenty-year-old who has strange sensory symptoms leading up to a headache, this unusual presentation of migraine is still much more likely than a stroke, which would be distinctly uncommon in someone this young. This doesn't mean that doctors should automatically jump to the common diagnoses, but it does help keep things in perspective.

#3. Good stories for uncommon conditions. Thinking about what *else* the story could represent is important, because it just might be that the story is classic for an uncommon condition. On first pass, a forty-year-old woman with no prior history who presents with crampy abdominal pain and nausea most likely has viral gastroenteritis. But say her symptoms are severe and come in distinct waves, and she has no diarrhea to speak of. Her story turns out to be less typical of gastroenteritis (a common condition), but it's classic for a more common condition: a twisting of her small intestines, which in some cases is a surgical emergency. Although rare, especially in someone of her age range with no prior surgeries, this disease matches her story, and the astute doctor would have recognized the pattern and considered this in the differential diagnosis.

#4. Not-so-good stories for uncommon conditions. For obvious reasons, this is the most difficult set of differential diagnoses to come up with. This is the list of true "zebras" because they are unusual presentations of uncommon diseases. Patients with diagnoses that fall into this category often go through years of uncertainty before the diagnosis is made. In retrospect, though, many aspects of the initial story don't fit anything else. When coming up with a list of differential diagnoses, this is an important category to keep in the back of the mind. Diagnoses in this category rarely come up in the first go-around, emphasizing the importance of asking again, "What *else* could it be? What *else* are we missing?"

"There are thousands of diseases out there," you may be wondering. "How can doctors consider every diagnosis and not go crazy?" One tip-off is if the story doesn't really fit any other diagnosis. That should be a sign to the doctor to keep looking—and for the patient, too.

As you tell your story, and certainly before the doctor walks out of the room, find out how your doctor is thinking about your diagnosis. Which of these four categories of differential diagnoses are they considering? Offer to think it through with them. Doctors may not know what you mean by Category #1 or #3, so ask them directly, "Would this be a common condition for someone like me? Would this be a usual presentation? Is there anything else that this could be, perhaps something less common?" and so forth. This is the type of process that builds your partnership and helps to ensure that your diagnosis is not missed.

Dr. Wen: One of the reasons to make sure patients and doctors work through the differential diagnosis together is that it allows doctors to address the diagnoses that their patients are most worried about. Almost every day, I'm surprised what I find out when I ask my patients the simple question: what do *you* think this could be?

A young lady who came in for dizziness and back pain admitted to me that she was most concerned about being pregnant. She hadn't been using contraception and she was late for her period. Pregnancy hadn't even occurred to me, yet when she voiced her concern, I knew immediately why she had sought medical care: her "chief complaint" was neither dizziness nor back pain, but concern for pregnancy.

A second-grader was brought in by his grandmother ostensibly for a

---

+ 911 ACTION TIP

Make sure your doctor shares her differential diagnosis with you. If the list seems short, keep on asking, "What *else* could this be?" Help your doctor come up with a thorough, if not exhaustive, differential diagnosis.

✚ 911 ACTION TIP

If the doctor doesn't ask what it is that you are the most worried about, bring it up yourself. It could significantly change your differential diagnosis, in addition to giving you the reassurance you need.

headache, but I puzzled at why he kept on saying his head felt fine. It wasn't until I asked the grandmother what she was worried about that she told me she had given him twice the amount of ibuprofen syrup that was recommended on the bottle and was actually worried about a toxic overdose. If she had accidentally poisoned her grandchild, how could she possibly explain it to his parents?

Tell your doctor what you're concerned about. Tell them that the reason you're worried about your palpitations is that you're scared of a heart attack, and that the reason you came in for your cough is that you're worried about cancer. Many people are afraid of the unknown; you don't know why you are having these new symptoms, and that's what is concerning you. Unless *your* "worst case" diagnosis is included in the differential diagnosis, you won't leave the doctor's office reassured—and worse yet—you may end up with the wrong diagnosis.

Dr. Kosowsky: In the process of going through the differential diagnosis with my patients, it's common that they will tell me something that completely changes how I was thinking. Sometimes this is what clinches their diagnosis. The other day, I had a young man come in with eye pain. His right eye was red and couldn't stop tearing. My resident had seen this patient first, and it seemed like a pretty straightforward case: the young man said he had "conjunctivitis"—an inflammation of the eye—in the past and that this felt the same. The diagnosis seemed to fit. He just wanted something to relieve his symptoms.

"Ah!" I said, "But remember that most of what's labeled conjunctivitis isn't actually conjunctivitis!"

The resident wasn't as excited. Neither was the patient. He had already been given a diagnosis—though when the resident and I went in to speak with him, he seemed unsatisfied. When I asked him what was the matter, he said, "So why do I always get conjunctivitis?"

"Well," I replied carefully, "there are a lot of different things that can cause conjunctivitis. Viruses, for example. But usually you'll have other viral symptoms along with it, like coughing, runny nose, sore throat." He shook his head. "And it's pretty contagious, so I usually hear about other family members or close contacts having something similar." No response. "Allergies can cause conjunctivitis," I continued. "But that tends to be extremely itchy and not so painful." Nope—it wasn't itchy in the least, and he'd never had allergies before. We went on to talk about other possibilities— trauma to the eye, prolonged contact lens use—nothing really fit.

I was pretty convinced by this point that "conjunctivitis" wasn't the correct diagnosis after all. "Hmm, perhaps it's time to expand our thinking. Let me ask you a question," I offered. "When you've had this before, has it always been in one eye?"

He thought for a moment. "Yes, as a matter of fact. And it's always the right eye."

"It's painful, right?"

"Unbelievably. I just don't like to complain."

Now we were onto something. "Tell me more about this pain. I'm beginning to think that may be the key to your diagnosis."

He proceeded to tell me about similar bouts of "conjunctivitis" every few months or so. Every "outbreak" was preceded by intense pain, always on the same side of his head—right behind the eye. He'd suffer through a day or two like this and then, magically, everything would be better.

My resident and I looked at each other, and at him. There it was, the diagnosis, staring straight at us. This man didn't have conjunctivitis; he had cluster headaches! Cluster headaches are characterized by severe pain on one side of the head or face, often just behind the eye. They are commonly accompanied by redness and tearing of the side on the affected side. The timing of his symptoms put cluster headache at the top of our list of differential diagnosis. This is a diagnosis that we wouldn't have even thought of had it not been for the patient's involvement in the process of coming up with his own differential diagnosis.

Later that day, the resident came up to me and asked how he could have

---

✚ 911 ACTION TIP

Your doctor should share her thinking with you. At every step of the process, feel free to ask, "What do you think I have? Can you please share it
with me?"

---

come to this diagnosis sooner. "I don't get it. He denied having headaches
when I asked him about earlier."

"Of course," I replied. "He's not a complainer, and anyway, he didn't
think of his pain as a headache—he thought of it as eye pain. If you really
want to figure out what's going on, you have to tell the patient what you're
thinking."

The same applies for the patient: make sure to ask your doctor what he
or she is thinking.

Partnering for the decision-making process

> The theories which I have expressed here, and which appear
> to you to be so chimerical, are really extremely practical—so
> practical that I depend upon them for my bread and cheese.
> —Sir Arthur Conan Doyle, *A Study in Scarlet*

We discussed the importance of sharing in the thought process and helping
the doctor to come up with the differential diagnosis. What happens next
is that the differential diagnoses needs to be narrowed down. One way to
do this is through a cookie-cutter pathway. By now, you know to be on the
lookout for these pathways that force you to do tests that aren't necessarily in
your best interest. What if your doctor recommends a particular test—how
do you know if it's useful or not? Well, a useful test is one where the results
are likely to impact the likelihood of one diagnosis over another. For example, if you suspect pregnancy, a pregnancy urine test can help to confirm
it, or if it is negative, to point in favor of other possibilities. Tests can also be
helpful to exclude certain diagnoses. A patient with coughing and fever

may benefit from a chest X-ray to exclude pneumonia before a diagnosis of bronchitis is made.

Unfortunately, many doctors see tests as just another part of the cookbook approach to diagnosis: if symptom A exists, then do test 1. If the result is X, then proceed with tests 2 and 3. Nothing could be further from the truth. This is why it is so critical that the next part of the process—choosing what tests (if any) to do—be a deliberate decision between patient and doctor.

Think back to your last doctor's visit. Did your doctor ask for your input as to what tests to do next? We took an informal poll of twenty of our nonphysician friends by asking them to think back to their last doctor's visit, and the answer was unanimous: no.

"The doctor said I was fine and I didn't need tests," some of them told us. Others said that their doctor informed them they needed some blood drawn and some kind of imaging study: an X-ray, an ultrasound, maybe a CT scan or MRI. Our friends were told that testing would help figure out what they have, but not often were they told what, specifically, the doctor was looking for.

In a true partnership, the patient is integrally involved in this important part of the diagnostic process. After all, patients can't really give consent to a test unless it's clear what the test is intended to show and how it may help get to a diagnosis. "We should send off for 'basic labs' " is not a justification for a test; nor is "a CT can help us figure out what you have." Instead, the doctor should be able to explain what the lab tests or CTs are looking for and how it will narrow the differential diagnosis or confirm the working diagnosis.[3]

Some lab tests are ordered almost reflexively. For example, a complete blood count that measures red and white blood cells and platelets is often considered part of "basic labs." There may be valid reasons to routinely check a patient's blood counts. Cancer patients, for example, have these measured all the time, because certain chemotherapies can cause dangerously low cell counts. Yet, many times, the blood count is checked in patients presenting with a variety of different complaints, simply because it is part of a pathway that involves "basic labs." But why obtain a test that's not necessary in the first place?

As we've discussed, no test is without risks. Take the ubiquitous CT scan. More and more studies are detailing the risk of radiation exposure; one study found that a single CT scan, in a healthy forty-year-old woman, confers an additional one in 200 chance of cancer over her lifetime—from that one CT scan alone.[3] Another study projected 29,000 excess cancers as a result of CT scans conducted just in 2007.[4] Most people would think twice about getting a CT scan with those odds. Yet, how often are patients counseled on the risk of radiation?

Instead, patients are simply told that they should get the CT because that's the "next step," with no discussion of risks and benefits. We believe that going ahead with a test just "to see what it shows" or "to make sure we don't find anything bad," or because some algorithm recommends it, isn't good enough. On the other hand, if there is a clear reason for the scan—for example, if the differential diagnosis points to bleeding spleen or ruptured appendix—the slight increase in a lifetime chance of cancer would be acceptable.[3]

Every test involves risks and benefits. We advocate for our patients to be involved in the diagnostic process, deciding which tests make sense and weighing (with the doctor) the risks and benefits. You should have the ability to ask questions, to understand what the test is likely to show and how it will (or won't) be helpful in making a diagnosis. You should find out if the test is part of a set pathway, and if so, challenge whether the pathway is right for you or not. You should be able to say no and discuss alternate strategies if the risks and benefits of the particular test don't make sense.

✚ 911 ACTION TIP

If your doctor says that a particular test is being done because it is part of a "set of labs," this could be a warning sign that you are being ushered down a pathway. Feel free to ask right out whether you are on a particular pathway to "rule out" or "work up" a particular illness, then request that you understand the doctor's thought process for what you *do* have instead of just what you don't.

Dr. Wen: One of the founders of emergency medicine, Dr. Greg Henry, has a great quote about CT scans: he calls them "the last refuge of the intellectually destitute." There's something very profound about this statement. CTs are an easy way out for doctors who don't talk to their patients or who don't want to think too hard about differential diagnosis. Some doctors order a scan because they think they are less likely to be sued for "missing" something. As Dr. Michael Weinstock, an emergency physician from Ohio likes to say, "This practice is akin to choosing long-term risk for the patient over short-term risk for the practitioner." That's not the kind of medicine I would want my doctor to practice on me.

Dr. Kosowsky: Another important thing to keep in mind about testing is that it often leads to further testing. Remember that tests are defined according to 95 percent of people who fall into the "normal" range, meaning that 5 percent of people who actually have no problems will end up being "abnormal" based on their test. We've seen how patients, like Annette with her incidental discovery of a "lung nodule," end up having procedures done because of incidental findings on a CT scan. When all was said and done, the finding was exactly that: incidental. And tests carry their own risks, not to mention the need for follow-up studies with additional radiation exposure and more lifetime risk of cancer—all because of something that wasn't dangerous to begin with.

Dr. Wen: Not to mention that the patient goes through months of worrying while the doctor is "working up" something that was never relevant to begin with. Pulitzer–winning journalist Nicholas Kristof wrote a column on how he was discovered, based on a CT scan, to have a cyst in his kidney.[6] He had the mass removed and was relieved to find out that it was benign—but not without first undergoing weeks of uncertainty, not to mention a painful surgery. The irony of his story is that the CT never had to happen in the first place. Renal cysts are almost always benign; in fact, nearly half of people over age fifty are estimated to have renal cysts.[7] However, once a cyst is discovered, it prompts further testing and invasive procedures that are ultimately unnecessary.

The prevalence of "incidentalomas" is the reason that medical and public health associations don't recommend routine screening X-rays or ultrasounds or CTs to diagnose malignancies, and why "total body MRIs" as advertised on billboards and TVs are a bad idea. Without a good reason for a particular test—without a carefully thought-out differential diagnosis—the CT or MRI may turn up all kinds of extraneous information that represents noise and not actual information.

Dr. Jerome Hoffman, a professor of medicine at the University of California, Los Angeles, famously talks about how, in an ideal world, studies would only focus on the thing that's being looked for. If appendicitis is the concern, the result of a test a doctor ordered should only include information about the appendix (or about something else that provides a better explanation for the acute problem). It shouldn't also describe an incidental lymph node or liver cyst, because these only confuse the picture, and invariably result in more tests and added anxiety.[8] In the real world, it's not really possible for doctors and patients to ignore the rest of the screen, so to speak, but his point mirrors ours: tests should not be ordered in a shotgun approach; rather, the only reason to order a test is if we have a specific question in mind and the test can help to answer that question.

As an interesting aside, Dr. Hoffman himself is (with a group of his colleagues) the pioneer of one of the most commonly-used "rules" in emergency medicine, the NEXUS decision instrument for ordering cervical c-spine X-rays after an injury.[9] He is also the first to say that rules like his are often applied and interpreted incorrectly. For one thing, rules are established on populations, not on individuals: they may work for "most" people between ages twenty and fifty, but not all—and you may be the exception. Also, rules typically have arbitrary cutoffs. Many rules, for example, use a specific age as a criterion, or heart rate. But does it make sense that someone who just turned 65 has to have an X-ray, but if their injury occurred last week, they were OK without one? Or that a patient with a heart rate of 99 beats per minute is fine, but if the heart rate goes up to 100, they suddenly need a blood test?

"Clinicians used to be taught to rely as much as possible on their clinical acumen to make decisions," Dr. Hoffman says. "Somehow we've gotten away from this, and have developed an irrational reverence of tests and rules. But

---

✚ 911 ACTION TIP

Any time your doctor recommends that you get a particular test, find out the risks and benefits of the test. If the risk sounds significant, ask whether it's necessary to get the test and what the alternatives are.

---

tests and rules don't make the diagnosis: doctors do. Doctors need to get a lot better at trusting their own judgment." He adds that "every decision instrument, including the ones my colleagues and I derived and validated, should contain a clause that talks about 'clinician gestalt,' which, in every case where there's a conflict, ultimately has to be allowed (in consultation with the patient) to trump whatever the rule tells you."

Tests are not inherently evil; when there is a specific rationale, they provide much useful information. A young woman with abdominal pain for a few hours that became more localized to the right lower quadrant pain might well have appendicitis, and the risk of delaying the diagnosis probably outweighs the risk of radiation from a CT scan.[10]

But what if the same young woman had been having intermittent abdominal pain for a year, associated with diarrhea and constipation, and has already seen multiple doctors for this pain? It certainly doesn't sound like acute appendicitis. Doing a CT on her would not be for any specific reason, other than that we just don't know what else is going on. That rationale just isn't good enough.

What if it's not the doctor, but the patient, who is demanding the test?

Dr. Wen: The other day, I had a patient, a young financial analyst in his mid-twenties, who insisted that he wanted a CT of his head. He'd been having headaches that were worse than his usual migraines. He admitted to being under a lot of stress and sleeping little, but refused to accept that his lifestyle could have been related to his headaches. "I need a scan, a CT, a MRI, whatever," he said. "I need to find out what's wrong."

Dr. Kosowsky: So what did you do?

Dr. Wen: I tried a lot of things! I explained to him about how head CTs are only good for finding certain things, like a hemorrhage, or a large tumor, or a buildup of fluid in the brain. I reassured him that we were quite confident from his history and physical exam that none of those things were likely. I talked to him about his stress at work, his worries about being fired, and how he was dealing with life in Boston now that he had just broken up with his long-term partner. I gently hinted, then more strongly stated, that the stress was the reason behind his headaches. Nothing seemed to make a difference.

Dr. Kosowsky: I bet I know what you did that worked: you made a deal with him.

Dr. Wen: That's right! How did you know?

Dr. Kosowsky: Because the fundamental component of the patient-doctor relationship is the partnership. That diagnostic partnership means doctors have to explain our thought process to patients; it also means that patients have to share their concerns with their doctors. Some patients come in asking for something very specific, and we have to decide whether or not it's a reasonable request.

Take antibiotics for a common cold. Now, we know that most upper respiratory infections are caused by viruses and that antibiotics don't help, but a lot of doctors give them out like candy. Why? Because the patients expect it. I don't think giving unnecessary medicine is good practice, but I do think that understanding a patient's expectations is an important step to building a partnership—and is actually an opportunity for education. So when my patients come in asking for a test or a prescription that I don't think they need, I tell them that I'll make a deal with them: they have to hear me out and I have to hear them out, and at the end, we'll make the decision together. Usually, after they've heard my spiel about how antibiotics won't help them feel any better but how they can have side effects, like diarrhea and yeast infections and potentially even very serious reactions, they don't want them anymore.

Are patients less satisfied with their care when doctors don't give them antibiotics? Actually, studies have shown just the opposite. Parents whose pediatricians did *not* give antibiotics for ear infections reported a higher degree of satisfaction with their care than those who were given antibiotics. After a discussion with their doctor about the risks and benefits of antibiotics, only 30 percent of parents given the option to fill the prescription actually did.[11] Researchers attributed this difference to the conversations that happened in the process of not giving antibiotics; by establishing a partnership and being explained the rationale of why a particular diagnosis was made and why a particular treatment was decided, patients gain more understanding and are more satisfied. Most patients don't go to the doctor wanting antibiotics or a CT scan, and even if they do, once they understand the risks, they quickly change their minds. What patients want is a diagnosis and a sensible treatment plan: a clear understanding of what they have and how to get getter. This is hardly a surprise; it's actually quite common sense.

Dr. Wen: Clear communication was exactly my aim with this young man who had headaches. I told him that we were going to start from the beginning and think through his diagnosis, and that at the end, it was his choice: if he still insisted on getting a head CT, we would do it. That was our deal. We reviewed the differential diagnosis of his headaches, the relative likelihood of various conditions, and why I was giving him the working diagnosis of tension headache. I explained to him some treatments for this, such as relaxation techniques, exercise, and counseling. We talked through his concerns. We both listened to each other, and in the end, I didn't have to say anything: he agreed that he didn't need a CT after all, and was going to try the treatment I recommended for his headache. I'm glad we were able to reach the decision together, and I think we both learned something in the process.

✚ 911 ACTION TIP

Always find out from your doctor exactly why she is recommending a particular test. What is the test looking for? Similarly, if you think you need a test, explain why, and use it as a starting point of your discussion for whether the test can help get you to your diagnosis.

Dr. Kosowsky: What if he had still insisted on the CT scan? What would you have done?

Dr. Wen: Interesting question. I think, in the end, if that's what my patient needed to be reassured that he was fine, I would have ordered the CT scan. To the extent that he was stressed out about the headaches, and the stress itself was exacerbating his headaches, a CT scan may even have been therapeutic! Our goal in this partnership approach is to involve our patients in the decision-making process and to empower them to make decisions based on what's right for them. Our goal is not to ration CT scans or to eliminate tests; we just want our tests to be used the right way, by doctors who know what they are for, and on patients who understand the benefits, risks, and limitations. We want to make sure that the doctors' goals and the patients' goals are always one and the same: to arrive at the diagnosis together.

---

911 REVIEW

- Before you consent to diagnostic tests, you need to go through your differential diagnosis with your doctor. You need a chance to understand it and to refine it.
- Tests can help to narrow the differential diagnosis to the working diagnosis, but there needs to be a clear rationale for every test done.
- You should understand the risks and benefits of each test, and to have a discussion on alternatives.

Twelve

It's Just Common Sense

You've told your story and highlighted the important features of the narrative. You became involved in the examination of your body. You've worked with your doctor to develop a differential diagnosis. And, perhaps aided by the results of some thoughtfully selected tests, you've narrowed down the differential diagnosis as far as you can. Now what?

Preventing misdiagnosis doesn't end here. As we have already seen, there are a number of pitfalls that could still result in a wrong or a missed diagnosis. Since diagnosis is the key to your care, you need to be sure your doctor gets it right. In this chapter, we provide suggestions for how to avoid some of these pitfalls and continue to remain in control of your healthcare.

Does the diagnosis make sense?

> Everything must be taken into account. If the fact will not
> fit the theory—let the theory go.
> —AGATHA CHRISTIE, *The Mysterious Affair at Styles*

When you go to the supermarket and the cashier is adding up your bill, what do you do? You might follow along and do the mental math in your head, cent by cent. Maybe you use the calculator on your smartphone. Or, like most of us, you wait for the final bill, then ask yourself, "Does that seem right?" If the amount is what was expected, you pay the bill, but if it's double or triple what you usually pay, you would take a second look, because what you see just doesn't make sense.

We perform this type of reality check in so many parts of our lives that it would seem to be a natural extension to apply it to our healthcare as well. First and foremost, always ask yourself, was I given a diagnosis? If not, what is going on? It may be that your doctor still hasn't come to any firm conclusions, but even if there is no definitive diagnosis, your doctor must have a working diagnosis—otherwise, on what basis could he make any decisions?

Something else to watch out for is if your final diagnosis sounds like a symptom (e.g., "chest pain" or "foot tingling"). Ask your doctor what that's supposed to mean. Does he really have no clue what could be causing your symptoms? Or does the doctor have some ideas, but since it's nothing serious, he's just not bothering to tell you? Does he think you may just be anxious, or a hypochondriac, but he doesn't want to say it to your face?

What if your doctor tells you that she is not sure? It's certainly possible that she doesn't know yet. Some diagnoses take months or years to confirm, and you wouldn't want your doctor to make up a diagnosis just to make you feel better. However, the doctor should give you some idea of what she thinks you have. Perhaps she gives you more than one working diagnoses.[1] This is OK. You should welcome this level of honesty, but should also make sure you have a plan for how you and your doctor will work toward a more definitive diagnosis.[2]

✚ 911 ACTION TIP

Watch out if your doctor gives you a diagnosis that sounds like a symptom. Ask your doctor for clarification.

✚ 911 ACTION TIP

Ask yourself: was I given at least a working diagnosis? If not, make sure you explicitly ask your doctor for one. If she says she is not sure, you must ask her to make a list of possible diagnoses and to come up with a plan for narrowing down the list.

Let's say that your doctor presents you with a working diagnosis. The next thing to do is to inquire about the natural history of that diagnosis. Disease processes tend to follow a typical course. A disease is not simply a snapshot in time or a list of symptoms, however carefully described. The natural history of disease has a beginning, a middle, and an end. It has twists and turns. Depending on the individual and the surrounding circumstances, the natural history of a particular disease may not have the same ending every time—in fact, it rarely does. But it's the key to understanding real-world diagnoses, and the first step to checking whether your diagnosis makes sense.

Let's take the common cold, a viral illness. We all know this: you start with runny nose, cough, and fever. You may have a sore throat, muscle aches, and generally feeling tired and run-down. These symptoms usually last two to three days, then you start feeling better. That's the natural history of a typical viral illness.

Patients who still feel terrible after a week, especially if they are still running fevers, probably have something other than a simple virus. We once saw a child who was supposed to have a "viral illness" for four weeks and ran temperatures to 104 every day until she had a seizure. Four weeks is far outside the normal natural history for this disease. Doctors know this, but patients need to know, too, so that they can challenge their doctor when the natural history doesn't fit their story, or come back to the doctor if their symptoms don't follow the expected course.[3]

Along the same lines, knowing the natural history can also be reassuring. We certainly see patients who are still coughing three or four weeks after a viral illness. Now, that seems like a long time to have symptoms—or is it? It turns out that persistent coughing after a viral illness is not all that uncommon. It's a diagnosis called postviral bronchitis, which is characterized by a dry cough that lasts after the initial viral symptoms go away. Knowing the natural history can help to reassure you that what you have is normal and okay.

Let's look at some other examples of common illnesses. Simple urinary tract infections may take a day or two to resolve. It's important that you know not to be disappointed if your symptoms don't suddenly disappear after your first dose of antibiotics.

Or muscle strains. After a minor car accident, we tell our patients that if their low back is sore, expect it to be worse the following day. That's the natural history of low back strain. Like the soreness you have after going to a gym for the first time in a while—it's always worse the next day. So we tell this to patients, and they know what to expect.

One more example: certain types of injuries are highly prone to infection, for example, puncture wounds.[4] When we are treating a patient with a puncture wound, we always mention this aspect of the natural history. This inevitably brings up some discussion about what to be on the lookout for (redness, swelling, etc.), what can be done to reduce the risk (keeping the wound dry, allowing the wound to drain), and whether there is any role for antibiotics (probably not). After all this discussion, patients are generally reassured, but more importantly, if they do end up with an infection they know when to seek medical care.

Of course, the natural history of the same disease won't look exactly alike for everyone. We talked before about how there are variations of diseases with typical and atypical presentations. This is another reason to have a discussion with your doctor about the typical symptoms and the usual natural history. If your symptoms start to seem less typical for the diagnosis that's being proposed, ask if they've seen cases of atypical presentations that are similar to yours. Inquire if there are other things on the differential diagnosis that may better explain your atypical presentation. Just because your doctor has made a presumptive diagnosis doesn't mean that the case is closed. A suspect in a murder case is innocent until proven guilty, right? You and your doctor should always be willing to reconsider other possibilities. Together, you can come up with a list of differential diagnosis with both usual and unusual presentations for common and uncommon diseases. This will allow you to revisit possibilities that you, thought were less likely previously, and even come up with new potential diagnoses—new culprits—altogether.

Just the other day, we saw a young woman who we initially gave a presumptive diagnosis of viral gastroenteritis, the common stomach flu. She was in her thirties, otherwise healthy, and she had what seemed like typical symptoms: vomiting, loose stools, abdominal pain with no real tenderness to palpation of her abdomen. She wasn't so convinced of the diagnosis, though, and kept on asking if this symptom or that symptom were typical. Viral gastroenteritis failed her reality check; she didn't want us to think she was a complainer, but she had never had such severe cramps. When she finally told us more about the pain, and how it kept coming back to her left side, it led us to consider that she might actually have kidney stones. Although we don't typically think of kidney stones causing gastrointestinal symptoms, a high degree of pain can lead to vomiting and even loose stools. Indeed, she had five large stones in her left kidney, two of which were so big they probably wouldn't have passed on their own. Though her symptoms themselves were a bit atypical for kidney stones, it was her reality check that pushed us to think beyond our initial working diagnosis and broaden our differential diagnosis.

Once you understand your diagnosis, you need to ask yourself if the diagnosis makes sense. Perhaps you have only heard about this condition from something you saw on TV or because your aunt had it years and

---

✚ 911 ACTION TIP

Always ask your doctor what is the natural history of the diagnosis you've been given. If the natural history includes symptoms that don't sound like what you have, ask whether your diagnosis is correct. Are there other diseases on the initial differential diagnosis that may better explain your symptoms?

years ago. Don't discount this exposure. You have enough information to perform your own reality check and to formulate questions for your doctor.

Dr. Wen: My mother was diagnosed with breast cancer when she was forty-nine, and fought it courageously for seven years. During that time, she saw her oncologist frequently. She always went with a list of symptoms, and to his credit, the oncologist was always good about giving her a working diagnosis of some kind. Still, though, she often called me to complain that she didn't understand the diagnosis and how her symptoms could possibly be attributed to it. For example, she went to her doctor once because her stomach was hurting. He thought it was due to constipation caused by her "medications," and asked her to take some stool softeners. She couldn't understand why—if her "medications" were the cause of her problems, why was he telling her to take more of them?

I knew what her doctor meant. He suspected her abdominal pain was due to constipation, which was caused by the pain medications she was on—but either he didn't explain this to her, or she didn't understand what he said. "So why didn't you ask the doctor about it?" I would ask.

She never had an answer to this, but I could guess the reason. Questioning her doctor just wasn't something she could bring herself to do, and no amount of cajoling on my part could get her to change her mind. That didn't mean she always agreed with the doctor; actually, she often disagreed, and wouldn't follow his treatment recommendations. Throughout the entire time she was ill, I didn't understand the logic, and attributed her reticence to her having come of age in China.

As a doctor, now, I see that my mother was hardly alone: many patients are genuinely afraid to challenge their doctors. And I don't mean challenge the doctor as in pick a fight with them, but even to ask basic questions. When I talk to patients about their diagnosis, they tend to nod and agree with almost anything I say. Sometimes, they'll ask a question or two; very infrequently does someone actually stop me and say, "Hmm, that doesn't sound quite right."

In speaking with patient advocates about this, it seems that many patients think they would be rude or presumptuous to question a diagnosis, especially since they think they know so little. It's quite the opposite: doctors

---

✚ 911 ACTION TIP

Speak up the moment you have a question, the moment you don't under-stand something that the doctor said. Don't let more time—and more op-portunity for misunderstanding—pass by.

---

should *want* our patients to ask questions and help us perform a final reality check! In my practice, I've taken to asking patients specifically if they think the diagnosis I had in mind makes sense to them, because it encourages them to bring up any concerns or questions. Not infrequently, these questions lead to a real breakthrough and really change their diagnosis and management.

One patient that I remember very well is a gentleman is in his mid-eighties, Mr. Sean Cotter. It was a typically busy day, and I had just finished sewing up someone's laceration and splinting another patient's broken arm. Mr. Cotter was sitting on a stretcher in the hallway with his right leg on a pillow.

There was a man next to him that I recognized as one the attending car-diologists in our hospital. He introduced himself; Mr. Cotter was his father, he told me. He was worried that his father had a broken ankle.

Broken ankle, that was pretty easy, I thought. Under the watchful gaze of the cardiologist-son, Mr. Cotter told me that he had fallen earlier that day, twisting his ankle. His ankle was visibly swollen and painful, and he had a small cut over his forehead where he struck his head against a cabinet. I told him that to begin with, we would do an X-ray to see if there was a fracture.

"That's what I thought," the cardiologist said. He turned to his father. "You'll be out of here in no time." He left to go return a page.

Mr. Cotter, though, did not seem as certain. He was scratching his head. "All that sounds good, but I have one question, doc."

I thought he was going to ask about what would happen if he did have a broken ankle, whether he would get surgery, and so forth.

"Of course," I said.

What he said next, I'll never forget. "There's something I can't really explain: why don't I remember how this happened?" Mr. Cotter proceeded to tell me that this was not his first fall. In fact, over the last month, he had fallen at least three times. Each time, he felt a flutter in his chest, then came to a few seconds later. The other times, he hadn't been injured and so didn't want to come to the hospital and worry his son about it.

My entire thought process changed. Now, I was worried about his heart rhythm, and indeed, the EKG confirmed that Mr. Cotter had a high-degree heart block. His heart had taken to beating so irregularly and so slowly that it caused him to pass out, and in the process, to fall and twist his ankle. He was admitted to the cardiac ICU and had a pacemaker implanted that day.

Now, heart block sounds scary and it truly can be a life-threatening condition, one that I (and his cardiologist-son) would have missed had the patient himself not been observant and insistent on his own reality check! And Mr. Cotter was completely right. A sprained ankle was one diagnosis, and it wasn't wrong, but it didn't explain the much bigger question of why he couldn't recall falling.

It is extremely important to ask yourself the question of "why?" Why did you fall? Why don't you remember? Sometimes the series of "why" questions leads from one diagnosis to another to another. This is another example of how you, the patient, need to help take control of the story-telling—and even if a diagnosis has already been made, to continue to ask questions.

Dr. Kosowsky: So far, we have told you stories that generally ended well. The worst that happened was that people got more tests than they needed; they had a delay to diagnosis; and some had additional complications because of it.

Now, let me tell you a different kind of story. A sad one, one that hits close to home. It's about a sixty-eight-year-old woman named Catherine Miller. Catherine had been pretty healthy throughout her life. She took no

---

✚ 911 ACTION TIP

Remember to ask "why." Why do you have the symptoms that you have? *If* they don't fit with the diagnosis you are given, why is that?

medications, and had just been to her doctor a month ago for a routine checkup and been given "a clean bill of health." She was a retired teacher and proud grandmother, who had recently decided to go back to school for her paramedic license so that she could volunteer in her hometown of Newton, Massachusetts.

One day, out of the blue, she began having a strange sensation of numbness and tingling in both arms. The sensation passed in a matter of minutes, and she didn't make much of it. A few days later, she had the sensation again. This time, she also felt light-headed, as if she was going to pass out. Once again, the symptoms resolved over a short time, but now she was worried. She called her daughter—Beth, a nurse—who agreed with her that these symptoms were concerning enough to call her doctor. She dutifully called her internist, who saw her in the office later that afternoon.

He listened to her story, examined her from head to toe, and performed an EKG in the office. Everything seemed normal. At the end of the office visit, her doctor seemed reassured. "I think I know what's going on," he told her. "Hypoglycemia. You have low blood sugar. Next time you have this sensation, drink some juice. You should feel better."

Catherine had enough knowledge of the medical field to know something about hypoglycemia. She had been on ambulance runs with diabetic patients who had taken too much insulin without eating and had gotten into trouble with low blood sugar. Typically it was a family member who would call for help, and when the ambulance crew arrived, the patient would be starting to come around, after having been given some juice or something else with sugar. Sometimes, the patient was so out of it that the only way to get their blood sugar up was to start an IV and give the sugar through the bloodstream. What she didn't recall ever seeing was a case of hypoglycemia where the symptoms just got better on their own. In addition, although she knew that hypoglycemia could present with a variety of symptoms, she didn't remember anything about numbness and tingling in the arms. On top of that, she wasn't diabetic or taking any medicine, like insulin, that would lower her blood sugars. So why would this be happening now?

She thought about asking all these questions to her doctor, but she knew he was busy—he had been kind enough to squeeze her in to his schedule that afternoon, but the waiting room was getting packed. She figured he must know what he was talking about. He had been her internist for years, and she trusted him.

The next morning, Catherine felt the same sensation coming on again. She called Beth, who urged her to drink some juice as she had been told. She drank some juice and felt a bit better.

Later that day, Beth came over to pick her up for dinner. She found a carton of orange juice on the counter and her mother on the sofa. She called out to her. There was no response. Catherine was dead.

I was at Catherine's funeral. There was no medical examiner, no autopsy, no diagnosis. What I do know is the story from Beth's perspective because she is the wife of one of my close friends. Needless to say, the family was shocked. How could a healthy woman suddenly die like this? Was her death related to the symptoms she'd been having, that she went to her doctor for? Could her death have been prevented?

We may never know the answers to these questions. If I have to guess, I'd say that perhaps Catherine had a heart attack or a massive stroke, and the symptoms she'd been having were warning signs. I don't bring up this story to blame her doctor for missing the diagnosis, and I certainly don't mean to blame Catherine or her family in any way. Beth and her husband will never know whether anything could have been done differently to change the ultimate outcome. They did consent to have me to share this story to help other patients and their families to be vigilant in performing their own reality check. The diagnosis of hypoglycemia unsettled both Catherine and Beth. Yet, despite being health professionals themselves, they didn't question the doctor. They—and we—urge you to, every time.

Not every missed diagnosis is as dramatic or unfortunate as this. No matter if your symptoms are a minor inconvenience or very troubling, remember that arriving at your diagnosis is the key—but it doesn't just stop there, because you must perform your own reality check. The benefit of having the Internet and other resources readily available is that patients can go home and find out all kinds of things about their diagnosis.[5] But you don't have to wait until then. While you're still in the ER or at the doctor's office, ask questions. Formulate questions based on what you think you know about the illness. If you have never heard of the diagnosis or don't know much

---

+ 911 ACTION TIP

Once you arrive at a diagnosis, perform your own reality check. Use the opportunity to ask your doctor as many questions as you can think of: what are the symptoms you should expect with that diagnosis? Do you have all of them, some of them, none of them—why or why not? Is there something about the diagnosis that doesn't sound right? Do not leave before making sure your diagnosis makes sense to you.

---

about it, ask about what symptoms you should expect with that diagnosis. If the doctor tells you something that doesn't fit with what you have, ask if that's unusual. Or, if what the doctor tells you doesn't explain all your symptoms, ask how that's possible—do these additional symptoms mean anything? While you have the doctor's ear, take the time to understand and potentially correct the diagnosis you're given.

Are you forcing the diagnosis to fit?

We balance probabilities and choose the most likely.
It is the scientific use of the imagination.
—SIR ARTHUR CONAN DOYLE, *The Hound of the Baskervilles*

Dr. Wen: When I was an intern, I had a patient, Linda Labo, who I was convinced had an inflammation of her pancreas—pancreatitis. She was in her fifties, and came to the hospital on many, many occasions with recurrent bouts of pancreatitis. In fact, on that particular day, the nursing triage note labeled her chief complaint in one word: *pancreatitis.* A senior resident had seen her and told me that the case was a straightforward case of pancreatitis. When I went into see Linda, she seemed convinced, too.

"I'm nauseous, my belly hurts, and I don't feel well. It's my pancreatitis," she told me. "I just need some fluids and something for pain and nausea." She seemed anxious and irritable.

As an intern, getting to the right diagnosis wasn't a sure thing by any stretch, and here was a woman who was literally telling me what she had.

We've talked about the dangers of using a chief complaint as your diagnosis; here's a patient using a diagnosis as her chief complaint!

At the time, I didn't see the danger in this. Instead, I breathed a sigh of relief. I can focus on her treatment and move on to my other patients! I took a brief history, performed a cursory exam, and told Ms. Labo that I agreed—she clearly had pancreatitis, and we would be admitting her to the hospital. I drew some basic labs and ordered her fluids and some medications for pain and nausea. I gave the hand-off to the internal medicine team that would be taking care of her in the hospital, and moved on.

The hospital was full that day so she stayed in the ER, waiting for an open bed upstairs. Thank goodness for that. Two hours later, I was called to her room because she was still vomiting, and her heart rate hadn't slowed down despite treatment for pain and dehydration. She seemed pale and a bit sweaty, so I inquired if her abdominal pain was worse. She couldn't really say. By that point, her labs had come back and, interestingly enough, her pancreatic enzyme levels were not elevated as would typically be seen with pancreatitis. I told my senior resident about this, but he wrote this off the fact that her pancreas was probably "burned out" from all the abuse, and that normal labs were not uncommon in patients with long-standing pancreatitis. I ordered some more nausea medicine and another liter of fluids and went about my other business.

It wasn't until an hour later, a good five hours after she first came to the ER, that I went back to check on her. She really looked bad now, sweaty and groaning in bed and saying that she was in a lot of pain. Where was her pain, I asked her. She pointed to her upper abdomen—basically her chest—and said, "It really hurts."

Yikes! Her chest hurt! Maybe she was having a heart attack! We did an emergent EKG, but it looked OK. Her cardiac enzymes looking for damage in her heart were fine, too. All the while the tests were being done, she continued to look worse. She was breathing at over forty times a minute and her heart rate went through the roof—160, 180, almost 200. She began to have a seizure and had to have a breathing tube be inserted because she couldn't breathe on her own.

What else could be happening? We knew that she had a long history of alcohol abuse—it's a common cause of pancreatitis—but she had gone through detox a few years back, and when I had asked her about it earlier, she told me she hadn't been drinking since then. I hadn't pressed her on it because her story seemed so clear to me of recurrent pancreatitis! In fact, we found out later that she had fallen off the wagon a few months prior, and she was back to drinking at least a pint of hard liquor every day. Four days ago, she decided it was time to cut the drinking so she just stopped cold turkey. The symptoms that she was having, including abdominal pain and nausea, were all due to acute alcohol withdrawal.

When I visited her in the ICU a few days later, she confirmed the story for me and told me that she thought it would make it easier for her to receive care if she just said she had pancreatitis. In the past, it always worked to get her to the hospital, and she wanted to get her pain and nausea controlled quickly. She hadn't wanted to talk about the drinking because she was embarrassed about it. She had known that the symptoms she had this time were different from her usual pancreatitis. I should have known, too, because, in fact, they were actually classic for alcohol withdrawal. She was getting worse and worse in front of me in the ER. And I had missed it.

Dr. Kosowsky: Nobody likes to admit they are wrong, but I think there's a lot of value to sharing and learning from each other's missed diagnoses.

I can tell that you feel very bad about your miss, but I guarantee you that all doctors have missed diagnoses like this. To start with, one of the errors you mentioned right up front is that of diagnostic momentum. We saw this in the case of Annette who everyone thought had a pulmonary embolism, remember? In this case, the nurse, the senior resident, even the patient herself, were fixated on pancreatitis, so you were, too. Given her history, pancreatitis might have been a reasonable working diagnosis, but we should always step back and see if there's another diagnosis we're missing. Would pancreatitis have fit her symptoms? Probably. But was there anything else that it could have been—gallbladder disease, perhaps, liver problems, heart problems, other toxins or withdrawal from substances? Anything the patient may not have wanted to tell us? That's why it's so important for doctors to go through the whole differential diagnosis, and for the patient to make sure that everything is taken into consideration.

You said yourself how important it was to really get the whole story.

Someone who visits the doctor many times for the same chief complaint should raise red flags, not only because it might mean doctors have missed something before (like the case of Eileen with her fifteen ER visits for an undiagnosed hernia), but also because healthcare providers tend to have their own biases when it comes these "frequent flyers." Just the word itself implies something negative: when we label a patient as a "frequent flyer," we are in some sense delegitimizing their reason for seeking medical care.

It's important for patients to be aware of her doctors' potential biases. Take patients with "chronic pain." Anyone who's ever worked in an ER will tell you that these patients can be the bane of our existence. Most patients with "chronic pain" are to some extent chemically dependent on narcotic medications, but they are not all "addicts" in a pejorative sense. Yes, sometimes these patients can come across as manipulative or demanding, but underlying it all is a level of frustration with a condition that defies easy solution. It's more difficult, but just as important, to get a full story in these situations—and for patients with chronic conditions to expect a fair hearing when they see a doctor.

I recently had a case of a young man who always came in with back pain. He had a history of IV heroin abuse, and multiple medical records made reference to his "narcotic-seeking" behavior. The resident, the nurse, everyone was ready to write him off and send him on his way, but he grabbed me and said something very important. He told me, I know it looks like I come in a lot with pain, but this time, my pain is different and here's how. It turned out that he had an infection of his spinal column—an epidural abscess—that required surgery to treat, and could have been fatal if missed. It took a lot for this young man to get through to us, but he did, in spite of whatever biases we had going in. The point is that all of our patients should feel empowered to share the entirety of their story, no matter who they are or what other conditions they may have.

All of this illustrates the importance of the doctor to be vigilant, but I think it also points to the critical role of the patient too. Imagine how different it would have been if Ms. Labo said at the beginning, this is not the same as my usual pancreatitis, and although I'm not sure what this is, I'm worried?

Mistakes happen when we anchor to one diagnosis and force everything

---

✚ 911 ACTION TIP

If you are someone who suffers from chronic symptoms, it helps to let your doctor know what has changed this time that is prompting you to seek care. Is the pain different? If so, how? Is it worse? Is it in a different location? If it is interfering with your daily activities, make sure to mention this, too, because it provides additional context for understanding your history.

---

to fit. When additional information doesn't seem to jibe, doctors and patients both should continue to question whether the working diagnosis was right to begin with.

Dr. Wen: Ms. Labo ended up doing fine and escaped long-term damage from my miss, but I've tried ever since then to think twice, three times, four times, even when it seems "clear" what the diagnosis is from the beginning, just to make sure I'm not anchoring and forcing the diagnosis to fit.

Actually, this may be one place where a "checklist" has a role.[6] Once the patient and doctor have worked together to come up with a working diagnosis, we should look together to see if there's anything we missed. Does the diagnosis explain everything in the history? Physical? Labs? Studies? Is there anything that we've missed? Taking this kind of "retrospective history" may just raise the right red flags to uncover critical information.

I've shared this story with a lot of my colleagues to help prevent them from making the similar mistakes with their patients. I hope that by sharing it with you, you can help your doctors to best help you. You may think that you don't know enough about medicine to understand what exactly the doctor is diagnosing you with. But you do. You can help by being on the lookout for things that that don't add up. You may have a sense that what you feel this time is different from before. You may even know what you *don't* have, because you had that diagnosis before and it feels very different. Be really careful when it seems that everyone is telling you that you have one thing, but there are still some pieces to the puzzle that don't fit. If your doctor

---

✚ 911 ACTION TIP

Perform a final check. Does the working diagnosis explain everything in your history? Physical exam? Tests? Be on the lookout for anything that doesn't seem to fit, and let your doctor know.

---

doesn't seem to see these odd pieces, point them out. Don't be afraid to speak up. The doctor may have many patients, but you have just you to worry about—so get it right.

Have the symptoms changed/progressed?

"You will not apply my precept," he said, shaking his head. "How often have I said to you that when you have eliminated the impossible, whatever remains, however improbable, must be the truth? We know that he did not come through the door, the window, or the chimney. We also know that he could not have been concealed in the room, as there is no concealment possible. When, then, did he come?"
—SIR ARTHUR CONAN DOYLE, *The Sign of the Four*

Symptoms change and evolve; new data emerges from test results; perhaps a new bit of history emerges from another source. Both doctors and patients need to reevaluate new information all the time and be willing to adjust the diagnosis accordingly.

One patient we saw together was Captain James McCausland. He is a former air force pilot and a self-proclaimed "food fiend." When he retired from the military, he decided to open up a restaurant near Boston. The restaurant is known around the area for its celebration of fine meat and wine pairings, and he himself continued to serve as the restaurant's head chef. A big burley man with a bald head and a large red beard, he was a recognizable presence in the area. In addition to owning his restaurant, he was quite active in his community, leading a citizen's anti-crime initiative, and holding a position on the city council.

Captain McCausland came to the ER because for the past day and a half, he had been having numbness in his feet. A few years earlier, he had been diagnosed with adult-onset diabetes and he was adjusting to his new life-style: walking more, staying away from refined sugars, and taking a pill each morning to help with his blood sugars. Overall, he was feeling better than he had in years, but the funny feeling in his feet was bothersome. Could it be the new walking shoes?

Or, perhaps it was his diabetes. If not for the rather sudden onset of these symptoms, this could have been a classic for a condition called "diabetic neuropathy," a slowly progressive type of nerve damage that is often seen in patients with diabetes. So classic, in fact, the doctors who saw him in the ER that day thought it was what he had and told him he needn't worry.

It was a busy day in the ER, and it took several hours before Captain McCausland was ultimately discharged, with instructions to see his primary care physician in a week. Right before he left, he mentioned to one of the residents that his feet were feeling heavy, almost as if he had to drag them to walk. However, the resident had observed him to be walking when he first arrived, so nothing much was made of this and he was sent on his way.

Four hours later, Captain McCausland was back. Unlike the last time, when he walked into the ER, this time he was in a wheelchair.

"My legs were getting so weak I could hardly stand up," he tells us. "I was going to go home to sleep it off, but my staff convinced me this wasn't so smart. I called a taxi and could barely walk to it; the waiters had to help me." By the time he arrived back at our hospital, he couldn't even step out of the cab. "My legs just totally gave out."

Captain McCausland didn't have diabetic neuropathy—he had a rapidly progressing and life-threatening illness called Guillain-Barré syndrome. Guillain-Barré is an autoimmune disease that is extremely rare (about one case in 100,000), but his symptoms were the textbook presentation for it: numbness, weakness, and ultimately paralysis starting in the legs and pro-gressing upward. The minor numbness was only a harbinger of what was to come. In Captain McCausland's case, the paralysis spread rapidly from his legs to his arms and chest, ultimately threatening his ability to breathe. Within just a few hours of returning to the ER, the captain was on a ventilator machine in the ICU. Had his colleagues not convinced him to return to the hospital and he had gone home instead, he probably would have stopped breathing and died.

Guillain-Barré is a relatively rare condition. Was it a mistake for the first team of doctors not to diagnose him with it the moment they saw him? Certainly the diagnosis of diabetic neuropathy is a far more common cause of numbness in his feet.[7] But then, at some point, he developed weakness. That should have been a clue that something new was brewing. "Foot drop" is not a typical symptom of diabetic neuropathy. Anytime new symptoms develop or existing symptoms progress, the diagnosis should be reexamined and reconsidered.

Communicating a change in symptoms, perhaps more so than other parts of the diagnostic process, needs to be the initiative of the patient. That's because only the patient can know and communicate what his or her symptoms are and how they have changed over time. The doctor's duty is to take care to listen and reevaluate, but it's the patient who needs to raise the concern.

You need to feel comfortable bringing up new or evolving symptoms, even when it feels like crying wolf. Often, the new or changing symptom may just represent the natural progression of the suspected disease process. Sometimes, though, these changes signify something far more concerning: a complication, a side effect of treatment, or a sign that the working diagnosis was wrong and that the real disease is something else. Stiff neck after a car accident with whiplash injury is typical—but double vision or incoordination is not, and could signal a rare condition like vertebral artery dissection (tear of the lining of the major artery that leads to your brain). Symptoms of viral gastroenteritis may continue for two or three days—but shouldn't progress to urinating blood (a sign of kidney problems) or jaundice (a sign of liver disease).

Dr. Kosowsky: A lot of ERs have developed observation units to keep patients for additional monitoring and testing. I like to use our observation unit for exactly this purpose: to *observe* them. The natural history of most conditions involves change over time. Symptoms progress, evolve, improve, etc., but rarely do they remain entirely static. Often it's the pattern of change—the dynamic features—that define a syndrome and suggest a particular diagnosis or other. Imagine if someone showed you a still picture from a favorite movie. Would you recognize it? Maybe or maybe not. It would depend a lot on how "classic" the scene was. Now imagine being shown a five-minute clip of a favorite movie. Odds are, you'll recognize it without any difficulty.

So I take advantage of this: if I'm unsure or want to confirm my working diagnosis, I keep my patients to observe them. For example, someone with chest pain due to angina (lack of blood flow to the heart) may get better or worse, but it's not a static condition. A patient with chest pain due to muscle strain tends to get better with anti-inflammatory medicines. And so forth.

Since I can't be there continuously "observing," I rely on my patients to do the observation, and I do so explicitly. I tell the patient with chest pain: the reason you are here, more important than the fancy monitoring equipment or the blood tests, is to keep track of your symptoms. We need to hear about any new chest discomfort or other symptoms that you may experience. Even if it's the kind of thing you've had before, or you wouldn't normally go to the doctor for, you need to tell us about it. In this way, not only does the patient understand the importance of observation, but also they are empowered to be part of the diagnostic process.

The assessment of new symptoms doesn't stop when you leave the hospital: you should be informed of what red flags to be on the lookout for and feel comfortable returning if and when these symptoms develop. This is simply common sense. If your car just got repaired and you continue to hear the same clunk every time you hit the brakes, or if a new smell develops after pulling out of the shop, you would go back to the mechanic. The same applies when you go to your doctor. Your doctor should tell you how to reassess your symptoms after you go home; but, it's up to you to make sure you know what to look for and to seek care if symptoms changed or progressed.

To that extent, make sure you ask your doctors all the questions you can

---

✚ 911 ACTION TIP

While you're in the hospital, be sure to tell your doctor if there is a change in your symptoms.

+ 911 ACTION TIP

Ask all the questions you can before you leave your doctor's care. In particular, understand as much as you can about your diagnosis, and what are the warning signs to watch out for. Don't hesitate to seek care again if new symptoms develop.

---

before you leave the office (or ER, or hospital). Ask them what you should expect over the coming hours, weeks, and months. Be clear about what warning signs to watch out for. Clarify how long it would take for any treatment to take effect and how to know if the treatment is working. Establish a time period for following up with them or another doctor. This is your time to gather all the information you can. Once you get home, you should continue to be vigilant, and do not be shy about raising a concern if things don't go as expected.

We have emphasized the importance of diagnosis for several reasons. The first is obvious: the wrong diagnosis can lead to unnecessary testing and useless treatment at best and catastrophic outcomes at worst.

Another reason that diagnosis is so important is that it is the first of many steps in the healing process. This, too, is common sense: you need to understand what disease you have before coming to terms with it and learning how to live with the symptoms. One of our female patients in her late twenties told us about how she went through eight years of anguish because of unremitting pelvic pain, getting addicted to painkillers and missing months of work, before someone actually provided a working diagnosis of endometriosis. This condition occurs when the cells lining the uterus deposit grow in other parts of the body, causing severe and often debilitating pain.

"The day I found out that what I had had a name, I felt like this huge burden was lifted off of me," she says. "That's because I could finally stop worrying about what I had and focus on moving on with my life."

We see patients who get tested over and over again for chest pain or dizziness. They are scared and worried every time. Having a doctor tell them,

"We don't think it's a heart attack or a stroke," isn't enough to make their concerns disappear. And yet, when doctors provide the same patient with a working diagnosis of fibromyalgia or anxiety or atypical migraine, the patients are already starting to feel better. Understanding the diagnosis is the first step to having control over uncomfortable and frightening symptoms.[8] Hundreds of studies in the psychology literature have demonstrated that people are happier when they feel in control of their lives, and that, conversely, loss of control leads to depression and helplessness.[9] This applies to medical care as well; studies have shown that across a spectrum of mental and physical illnesses, patients do better with their treatments if they understand and are involved in the decision-making process.[10]

So why don't doctors provide a diagnosis more often? A good portion of the blame falls on the cookbook mentality that favors "rule-outs" over diagnoses, but there is also a component of psychology at work as well: many doctors want to be 100 percent certain before offering a diagnosis.[11] On the other hand, we have found that patients, by and large, are willing to accept some uncertainty in diagnosis. Patients want doctors to be open with them and to hear the truth. They are happy to share in the thought process to narrow the differential diagnosis to a working diagnosis, and they are willing to accept the uncertainty that the working diagnosis may not be 100 percent correct. At least there is something to go on, not just a list of things that they don't have, and they can develop a plan for moving forward and getting better.

This is why we emphasize the importance of partnership with your doctor to reach the working diagnosis. Patients have been conditioned to be satisfied if they walk away from an encounter with their doctor with a prescription, or a referral for additional testing or consultation. But that's not the only thing you need to walk away with. We urge you never to leave the ER, the clinic, or your doctor's office without a working diagnosis. And along with whatever next steps are advised as far as testing and treatment, you should be given an idea of what to expect if all goes well, and what to expect if it doesn't.

One of our heroes, the Nobel–prize-winner, humanist, and cardiologist Dr. Bernard Lown[12] likes to tell the story of how he went to an international conference and met a rather large Eastern European woman who was dressed in garish and what he thought was inappropriate clothing. Who is this woman at this conference of doctors and humanists? he grumbled to himself.

Among questions posed at the conference was, what makes a doctor a good doctor? This woman raised her hand and answered that a doctor is someone who makes you feel better after having seen them. Dr. Lown said that at that moment, he realized that she must be a doctor. A real doctor. A good doctor.[13]

You go to the doctor because you want to know what's going on and because you want to feel better. Your diagnosis is central to both of these. You deserve to find out what you have, and you should be involved every step of the way in partnership with your doctor, from telling your story to participating in your physical exam, to thinking through your differential diagnosis, to arriving at a working diagnosis. This is not too much to ask. You are the key to your own health, and you have to help your doctor help you.

911 REVIEW

- Diagnosis is the most important part of your care, without which you cannot begin to feel better. Don't leave your doctor's care without at least a working diagnosis.
- Perform your own reality check. Don't force your symptoms to fit a diagnosis you've been told.
- Find out what to watch out for. Report changes in your symptoms or any new concerns.

Part IV

How to Get to the
Right Diagnosis

Part III focused on the theory behind avoiding misdiagnosis, illustrated by cases from the ER and highlighted by the ✚ 911 Action Tips. Here in Part IV, we present the practical application of these concepts. Chapter 13 organizes the principles from Part III into the 8 Pillars to Better Diagnosis. Then, in Chapter 14, we provide "Prescriptions for Patients": how you can use the Pillars to radically improve your medical care. Chapter 15 illustrates how the application of the Pillars and Prescriptions works in practice by revisiting the four cases from Part II.

Thirteen

The 8 Pillars to Better Diagnosis

Mrs. Fiona McCloskey is a tough old cookie. That's according to her. Her three sons, all in their thirties, are not about to disagree.

"When Momma wants something, she'll get it done, you can bet on that," said her oldest son, a navy lieutenant. "She's not gonna back down for anybody."

Born to Irish immigrants, Mrs. McCloskey was a public school teacher in some of the roughest areas of South Boston for almost forty years. Her dream was always to move to Florida and live on a boat, and after she retired and her second husband died, she decided to do just that.

The first time she came back to Boston after the move, she ended up in the hospital for two weeks.

"Tells ya something, doesn't it?" she says as she leans back in her recliner, sipping a Long Island iced tea.

To be fair, she does acknowledge that her symptoms started when she was still in Florida. She had joined a senior theater production of *West Side Story*, and some of the other actors were coming down with colds. She started with some coughing and chills the day that she flew to Boston. Instead of feeling better after settling in at her eldest son's place, her troubled breathing only got worse, and two days after she arrived, she woke up feeling miserable.

Her sons brought her to the local ER. There, the doctors began to do "all kinds of tests" on her. She got a chest X-ray, EKG, and lots of blood work. She was told that she had to stay in the hospital because they were worried about her heart. So she got a CT scan of her chest and an echocardiogram, an advanced ultrasound, of her heart. They said they had to do a catheterization, where they looked at each of the vessels in the heart to see if there were any blockages. The catheterization was pretty much normal, but then her blood counts dropped because she had a bad reaction to one of the medications they used. She began bleeding from the area where they had done the catheterization and had to stay in bed for another day. When she got out of bed, she was so weak she couldn't walk. It took five more days before she was well enough to leave the hospital.

Mrs. McCloskey shakes her head when she recalls her hospital course. "I knew what I had: I had some kind of flu. It was bad, sure, but I knew there was nothing wrong with my heart."

It turned out that she was right; her heart studies were all normal. But why didn't she tell her doctors of what she had suspected?

"Because it's not my place to," she answers. "The doctors know what they're doing. I don't want to second-guess them. Besides, nobody wants to know what I think. I'm not the expert here."

So did that mean that she was satisfied with the care the she received? Her sons guffawed at the suggestion.

"All she ever did was complain to us," said the oldest. "But when the doctor came in and said, do this, this is the plan for you, she didn't say a peep."

"Momma would have stood up to anyone, but she just doesn't stand up to her doctors," added one of the younger sons. "She was like that when Pops was in the hospital, too."

In our experience, Mrs. McCloskey is like a lot of patients we encounter. People who wouldn't blink an eye when they're speaking up to their child's teacher or complaining about their utility bill become quiet and deferential when it comes to their healthcare. Successful businessmen and high-powered attorneys who are used to being leaders in every other arena come to the doctor's office and suddenly transform into acquiescent followers. "Tough old cookies" turn into "wallflowers" when it comes to their doctor.

It's no mystery why this happens. For one thing, there is a perceived information gap between what the patient knows and what they assume the doctor knows; the reason doctors go to medical school, after all, is to become experts. Patients also understand that doctors are busy, and they don't want to be seen as a burden to their doctors. No one wants to be seen as the "difficult patient."[1] In the end, patients end up putting far too much faith in the doctor's opinion and far too little in their own, to the effect that they question the value of their own input.

In our interviews with patients for this book, we've heard a number of variations that are surprisingly similar to Mrs. McCloskey's response.

"I only know one mantra for when I go to the doctor: KMS," said one person, a partner in a major accounting firm. "Keep Mouth Shut."

The origin of this mentality isn't hard to trace. Medicine has always harbored some paternalism: traditionally, the doctor was always the one who dispensed the knowledge and the patient was the one who accepted their wisdom. The difference, though, is that the doctors in days past had to listen closely to their patients to arrive at a diagnosis. Nowadays, doctors fall back on cookbook recipes and high-tech testing, rather than engaging with their patients in a personalized way. The consequence is that patients often have no choice but to take initiative and advocate for their own health. To "KMS" is to accept potential misdiagnosis and unnecessary tests.

To be sure, we have had patients who are "difficult" in every sense of the word: rude, obnoxious, and manipulative. Down the hall from Mrs. McCloskey on the cardiac floor was a gentleman named Benjamin Bender. Or, as he insisted on being called, *Doctor* Bender. Dr. Bender was a retired orthopedist who had his own theories about what made him sick, and made frequent adjustments to his own medications. He tolerated no differences of opinion, to the point that he would ask his wife to come to the hospital to fill prescriptions that he wrote for himself. Nurses and doctors alike avoided his room because he was prone to throwing objects at them when he disagreed with what they said.

In truth, "difficult patients" like Dr. Bender are few and far between. There is a vast difference between being engaged and being overbearing. You do not need to stay quiet to be a "good" patient; there is a way to be assertive and speak your mind, while at the same time respecting the doctors' expertise and acknowledging their suggestions.

We know that being an active participant every step along the way is the key to avoiding misdiagnosis. But how, exactly, do you actually advocate for yourself, especially when you are sick and have a pressing problem to address? In the last section, you saw some examples of what you can do when you are seeing your doctor to establish a partnership and become an active participant in your own healthcare. In this chapter, we organize the pitfalls and suggestions into the 8 Pillars to Better Diagnosis.

How on earth can I remember 8 Pillars, you may ask. Especially because the times I would use these are when I'm sick—or when a loved one is sick! This is why we believe in practice and preparation. You need to learn and practice the 8 Pillars now so that you will be prepared when you have to use them.

Be warned: learning the 8 Pillars is not going to be easy. Most of us have always thought of receiving medical care as a passive process that it takes time to change our mind-set to put ourselves in the driver's seat. At your own pace, we encourage you to read the Prescriptions for Patients in Chapter 14 as well as Appendix 2, which contains twenty-one exercises for practicing the 8 Pillars now so that you will be prepared for your next ER visit, doctor's checkup, or hospital stay. Appendix 3 contains two sets of worksheets that further help you organize your story. The Prescriptions give you tangible how-tos, and the exercises should help build confidence and provide guidance for when you or your loved ones need the right diagnosis and the right medical care.

Pillar #1: Tell your whole story

The story forms the foundation of diagnosis. Telling it may seem like an uphill battle, because the doctor, nurse, and tech may all be trying to steer away from a narrative and toward the cookbook world of "chief complaints" and close-ended questions. However, it is critical that you insist on telling your story. Work on becoming a better storyteller, and make sure that your doctor listens to and understands your whole story.

Pillar #2: Assert yourself in the doctor's thought process

Your doctor is thinking about something while she's with you. Assert yourself in her thought process early on. Find out what your doctor is thinking as she is listening to your history. Let her know that you want to be integrally involved in coming up with your diagnosis and in every step of your care.

Pillar #3: Participate in your physical exam

Participating in the physical exam is an excellent way to establish rapport and partnership, and for you to better understand your own body. As your doctor examines you, ask him what he is looking for. Make sure you understand the meaning of abnormal findings. Clarify how the findings confirm (or not) your doctor's thought process.

Pillar #4: Make the differential diagnosis together

Make sure that your doctor comes up with a thorough differential diagnosis. Decide, together with your doctor, how exhaustive your list needs to be. Keep on asking what *else* could be going on. Evaluate, together, the relative likelihood of each diagnosis on this list.

Pillar #5: Partner for the decision-making process

Once the differential diagnosis is generated, continue to partner with your doctor to devise a plan for narrowing down the list of possible diagnoses. Understand why certain diagnoses are being eliminated. Come up with a strategy to arrive at, at least, a working diagnosis. Determine, together with your doctor, how important it is to reach a definitive diagnosis.

Pillar #6: Apply tests rationally

Part of the decision-making process is to figure out, together with your doctor, what (if any) tests should be ordered to narrow down the differential diagnosis or confirm the working diagnosis. Do not just consent to tests; ensure that your doctor explains why each test should be done, what the risks and benefits are for the test, and what are alternatives to the test. Look out for cookie-cutter "pathways" and ask your doctor to tailor an approach just for you.

Pillar #7: Use common sense to confirm the working diagnosis

You should reach at least a working diagnosis at the end of every visit to the doctor. Before you leave, make sure that the diagnosis makes sense. Do a common sense check. If reaching a diagnosis is like putting together a giant jigsaw puzzle, check to make sure that what you have put together looks reasonable. Are any pieces missing? Are there extra pieces that don't fit? If the picture doesn't add up, go back to the drawing board to come up with alternate diagnoses.

Pillar #8: Integrate diagnosis into the healing process

A working diagnosis is a prerequisite for healing. Once you have a diagnosis, find out as much as you can about it. Look it up yourself. Discuss it with your friends and family. And ask your doctor questions: What is the natural course of the illness? What should I expect with this illness? What if our working diagnosis is actually wrong; what are the warning signs? What should I be watching out for? What treatment choices do I have, and what are the risks and benefits?

The mortar on which all these pillars are built is communication. You need to speak up and be your own best advocates. Throughout the book, we have seen examples of strong, professional woman and men like Fiona McCloskey and Arthur Coates who are outspoken in every aspect of their lives, except when it comes to their own medical care. Many articles have been written on how trying to be the "good" patient and keeping your mouth shut actually leads to inferior care.[2] Medical care is not a popularity contest. If you don't think your doctor understands you; if you don't think your story is being heard; if you don't agree with a part of your care; if you have questions that are not being answered—this is a problem, and you have to be the one to address it.

Internist doctor Lisa Sanders, of *House, M.D.* and *The New York Times*, says that patients are amazed when she tells them they often have to be the ones to put pressure on their doctors to make sure they are understood. "There are all kinds of pressures on doctors these days, to see patients faster, to use cookbook recipes, whatever the case might be—but that's not your problem," she says. "If you feel like your doctor is rushing through your history and isn't listening to you, tell him that. If you feel like you're just a number and your diagnosis doesn't matter, tell him that. It's the doctor's job to help you." In her experience, and in ours, doctors appreciate the frankness, especially because it is your advocacy that will lead to getting your diagnosis right.

Incorporating the 8 Pillars to Better Diagnosis into your life will be as much an adjustment for your doctor as it will for you. Initial reactions from doctors may range from puzzlement to outright resistance. Don't be discouraged; keep in mind that the age-old aphorism that practice makes perfect applies to the 8 Pillars to Better Diagnosis as much as it does for learning a new language or picking up a new sport. If anything, it may be even more difficult, because it requires a significant shift in mentality, on your part and on your doctor's. One thing is for sure: your actions will be noticed and they will have an impact. Practice the prescriptions and try the exercises now, before you are sick and subject to misdiagnoses and unnecessary tests, like Mrs. McCloskey.

911 REVIEW

- Your healthcare crisis is not the time to "keep mouth shut"; it's the most important time to speak up and be your own advocate.
- The 8 Pillars to Better Diagnosis provide a proven, step-wise strategy for you to advocate for your health.
- Practice the 8 Pillars today—before you get sick.

Fourteen

Prescriptions for Patients

Jessica Papin is a writer and literary agent with a particular interest in medicine and health. Recently, she had a terrible scare. It was her birthday, and she decided to celebrate by taking her family and close friends out on the Hudson River on an old-fashioned schooner. It was a very hot day, a day with "little breeze to speak of and even less shade." A dear family friend, who is seventy-seven, went below the deck to look at the crew's quarters with Jessica's nine-year-old niece. When Mrs. Ware emerged, Jessica thought that she looked odd. She was staring blankly into space and didn't respond when Jessica spoke to her.

Something wasn't right. "Mrs. Ware, are you OK?" Jessica asked again, touching her friend's face. "Do you want something to drink?"

Mrs. Ware stared straight ahead. Her eyes looked glazed, and she reached out as if to steady herself—except she didn't hold on to anything and slid down to the ground. Jessica called for help. People brought ice packs and water bottles and pressed them to Mrs. Ware's face. Within a few minutes, she began to respond and was able to say who she was, but still appeared confused about where she was and what she was doing there. She continued to have no recollection of what had just happened.

There was no doctor on board, and by the time the boat reached shore,

Mrs. Ware was back to her old self. She didn't want to go to the hospital, but Jessica insisted. "I thought I had done her in! Maybe she was just dehydrated and overheated, but what if this were a stroke?"

When they got to the doctor, Mrs. Ware was able to relay some of what had happened, but kept on turning to Jessica to fill in the details. What exactly happened again? What did she look like when she couldn't respond? How long did it take her to snap out of it? What other medical problems did she have again?

"The more she turned to me, the more I began to feel just as lost as she did," Jessica says. "I knew there was very limited time for us to convey what had happened to the doctor. The sequence of events started blending together. I didn't know the level of detail that I needed to go into. Was it relevant that she went below deck and that it was a hot day? Probably. What about that she ate lasagna for lunch, when everyone else ate seafood? Maybe. . . . Well, what about her high blood pressure and the fact that she recently switched to a new medication? Or that she had gained ten pounds, and was exercising less than she should (she has been a devoted aquacizer for years)? That she had successful double knee replacement surgery two years ago and recovered like a champ? That her father had bypass surgery in his late sixties and lived to be ninety? That she is the de facto primary caretaker for her three granddaughters, and hence, under a fair amount of stress?

"I've always thought of myself as being pretty knowledgeable about medicine, at least from the consumer's perspective, and pretty good at relating facts to doctors. I'm maybe one of few patients who's not afraid to speak up and interrupt the doctor and say, hold on here, let's start over. But I still felt like I didn't know how to approach the medical encounter. How much or how little should I have said? How could I have helped my friend convey her story? My guess is that many patients and their families wrestle with these questions."

In this chapter, we present Prescriptions for Patients to show exactly how patients—and their families—can apply the 8 Pillars to Better Diagnosis. Each Prescription starts with a patient's question, and we provide practical answers to demonstrate what you can do in the ER, hospital, or doctor's office. As before, important action tips are highlighted using the ✚ symbol.

In addition, we include two worksheets in Appendix 3 that we encourage you to make copies of and complete to help you apply the 8 Pillars. There is a one-page basic worksheet and a two-page in-depth one for when you have more time. You can supply them when you are ill or when your loved one or friend is the patient, and you, like Jessica, have to help them convey the story.

As you read on, think about a recent time that you or a loved one has been ill. Practice the Prescriptions. Try completing the worksheets; notice how much more empowered you feel to advocate for your own health.

Pillar #1: Tell your whole story

"What should I do if the doctor is fixated on my 'chief complaint'? I must have mentioned chest pain to the nurse at some point, because when I finally got to see the doctor, all he wanted to do was ask me questions about my heart. What I was really concerned about was the cough that hadn't gone away for two weeks, and whether I might have pneumonia!"
We have several suggestions:

✦ *Use your own words to tell the story.* Don't let someone else put words in your mouth. If what you have is a cough with chest congestion, describe what that feels like. Don't say you have "chest pain" just because someone else said you did.

✦ *Tell your story the way you would to a friend or family member.* Include details that are important to you, not just those that you think might be important for the doctor to hear. Allow the doctor to get to know a bit about you by describing your symptoms in terms of how they impact your daily life.

✦ *Make sure you communicate what is most worrisome to you.* What symptom most concerned you and why? Talk about why that particular issue brought you in on the particular day. This often helps the doctor think outside the box of what she determined ahead of time to be the chief complaint.

✦ *Start over.* If the message is still not getting through, ask to start from the beginning. "I'm not having chest pain—but I have been coughing a lot. Can we start at the beginning and talk about my cough?"

"When I go to the doctor, I often find myself boxed in by all the yes or no questions. How can I get to the 'how' and 'why'?"

✚ **Ask your own questions.** If you're posed a series of yes-or-no questions, it's OK to answer, but also go on to explain your answers in more detail to fully convey your story. If you don't understand why a particular question is relevant to your situation, ask about it. You may be surprised to find that the doctor himself doesn't know and is only asking the question out of habit. On the other hand, you may find out that issues you wouldn't have thought were related might actually be very important to tease out.

✚ **Interrupt when interrupted.** If your doctor cuts you off when you try to explain your answer as a "how" and "why," feel free to interject. Pretend you're having a conversation, even when it feels like you're being interrogated. For example, if you're asked "When did the headache start?" rather than responding "9:30 A.M.," go ahead and tell your story of how the pain started: "I woke up this morning and I was fine, then I started walking to work and the pain came on suddenly like a lightning bolt striking me." This is not a new tactic; a good attorney will often coach her client in advance to answer yes-or-no questions with a narrative so that answers can't be taken out of context. Interrupting is a way to ensure that your entire answer is heard, not just the part that the doctor thinks he wants to hear.

"But I'm going to be perceived as a bad patient! How can I possibly interrupt the conversation without having the doctor be upset with me?"

The majority of doctors will be happy, relieved even, if you interject with details that help them arrive at the correct diagnosis. Patients know their bodies and their stories the best; a good doctor will know this and will actively listen for your input.

There will always be doctors who persist in asking close-ended questions. What you can do in these cases is to ✚ **answer their pressing questions first.** If they want you to describe the location of your chest pain, describe it ("it's in the middle of my chest, right here"). If they want to know what you took to make it better, tell them ("I took an aspirin. It didn't help"). ✚ **Attach a narrative response at the end of these close-ended** *questions* ("it's in the middle of my chest, right here, and it started after I really pushed myself in swimming tonight").

If you feel like you are not being heard, ✚ *interject*: "Excuse me, doctor, I have tried my best to answer all your questions, but I am still not certain you've heard the whole story. Can you please help me understand why it is that I have been feeling fatigued and short of breath for the last two weeks?" and so on. You can take charge of the conversation at that point. It's your body and your duty to advocate for yourself if you don't feel like your story has been understood.

It is always important to ✚ *make sure you are courteous and respectful to your doctor.* Your doctor is a professional, and is probably trying her best to help you. You have a need to be heard and to tell your story, but make sure you present your point in a respectful manner. This will ensure that a good working relationship is present, and is critical to the active partnership you need to establish.

"I can't speak to a doctor like that! How can I get my doctor to really hear me out?"

Implicit in your statement is that you are somehow inconveniencing the doctor by asking them to hear you out. This not the case! In a medical encounter, you are the customer. The doctor is there to serve you, and her duty is to help *you*. It's not your problem if the doctor is busy and has other patients to see. You need to make it a priority that your story is heard.

The next time you feel like your doctor is not really listening to you, or is asking all the wrong questions, or is trying to go down a path that doesn't make sense to you, ✚ *speak up*. We recommend that you look your doctor in the eye and say, "Doctor, if you don't mind, I want to go back to what you asked me earlier about when the symptoms started." ✚ *Use clear and direct language*. State your point that there's something else you want to say, then proceed to tell your story and confirm that you are being heard along the way.

Another technique is to ✚ *redirect the conversation with clarifying questions*. For example, ask your doctor what he thinks about a particular symptom. If their understanding of the problem doesn't jibe with what you've been trying to tell them, let them know: "Actually, that's not what happened. First I started having trouble swallowing, then the pain in my chest began."

A good doctor will always try and summarize his understanding of the patient's history, but not all doctors do this or do this well. If your doctor does not present this for you, **+ ask for the doctor's summary of what you said.** "I just want to make sure we are on the same page," you can say. "Can you summarize for me what my story is and where we go from here?"

Many doctors have been conditioned out of listening, but you have the power to make a difference. Your active engagement will lead to better care for yourself, and for other patients that this doctor will see.

"I totally relate to Jessica's story. When I'm at the doctor, I can't remember all the things that are on my mind, and I have no idea where to begin. How can I sort through everything and figure what's important for the doctor to know?"

Figuring out what's important (and what's not) can be very challenging. Medical students spend years learning how to recount patient histories to their supervisors. You have to practice doing this. Focus on the following tips.

+ Start at the beginning and proceed chronologically. It helps the doctor to understand your story if you tell it in a chronological order. **+ Use concepts such as timing, pace, onset of symptoms, severity, changes over time—** these are key to arriving at your diagnosis, and will come through naturally if you tell your story from the beginning. Remember that all diagnoses have a natural history, and the better the chronology of your story, the better the fit can be.[1]

+ Draw it out. Our detailed worksheet includes a graph of symptom severity over time. You can use this graph to plot a symptom and how it has changed over time. Your horizontal axis can be any time interval you choose (hours, days, or months, depending on your symptoms). The vertical axis is your level of pain or discomfort. You can think of it on a scale of 1 to 10, with 1 being minimal pain and 10 being the worst pain, or just as "not so bad," "bad," and "very bad." If there are two or more symptoms of concern, you can plot them alongside each other. We provide some examples below:

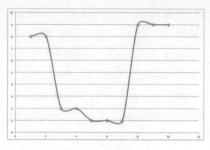

Pain was really bad, then it got better, then it came back.

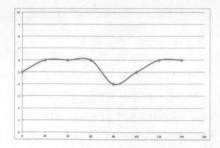

Pain stayed really bad so I finally decided to get it checked out.

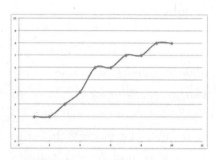

The pain just kept getting worse and worse.

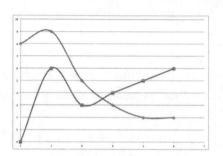

As the pain got worse, I got nauseous. After I vomited, the pain was better but I still felt nauseous.

✚ Provide your doctor with context and *tie the chronology to other events.* Instead of getting bogged down with exact times and dates, try to relate your symptoms to things that were going on in your daily life. Don't just say, "My headache started at 10:30 A.M."; instead, relate the symptom to what you were doing. "I first noticed the headache after a long day at the office," or "I felt the stomach cramps for the first time after getting home form the church picnic, but they went away after I threw up." Talking about details like this may seem extraneous, but understanding the context can help you and your doctor put together the temporal relationships of symptoms and identify factors that make your symptoms better or worse.

Related to the concept of context, it's more important to **✚ describe how your symptoms have impacted your life** as opposed to trying to quantify your symptoms in some random "objective" way. Telling the doctor, "My headache was so bad I had to leave work early for the first time in five years," is going to be more helpful than "the pain was a 9 out of 10." Mentioning whether you have had to miss school or work is another measure of severity. Explaining the impact on your daily life also gives your doctor a window to who you are, and improves the chances of the doctor making the right diagnosis.

+ *If something about your symptoms surprised you, emphasize it.* All good stories are driven by the element of surprise. "I thought I was just having a garden-variety headache, like the migraines I always have. Then, all of a sudden, the room started spinning and I couldn't stand up straight. That's never happened before!" Relating what surprised you will help make sure the doctor pays attention to this part and address it. And who knows; it might surprise your doctor, too, and completely change his thought process.

+ *Share your impressions with your doctor as you go along.* We all experience minor ailments from time to time and we do a pretty good job at making our own diagnoses. Accurate or not, these impressions are very important for the doctor to understand as he or she hears your story. For example, you might say, "At first I thought it was just a pulled muscle, because I had been working out with a new bench-press machine earlier in the week. But when the pain began shooting down my left arm I started to get worried." Or, "It feels like every other migraine I've ever had, it's just that it hasn't gotten better, and now my right eye vision is kind of blurry, something that's never happened before with my migraines." If your impression changed along the way, or if there are things that you think are *not* the cause of your symptoms, it helps to share these as well.

+ *Use simple language.* When you describe your symptoms to the doctor, don't incorporate medical terms unnecessarily. Patients often think it helps to talk in "medicalese," but this can lead you into trouble. If you have a fluttering sensation in your chest, explain how it feels; using the term *palpitations* may focus the doctor on your heart, but this may or may not be the issue. If you feel off balance, describe what it's like for you; saying that you have "vertigo" may lead your doctor down the wrong path. As much as you hear doctors using these terms, try to avoid saying things like "intermittent," "radiating," or "associated with." Don't be shy to tell your doctor what you think is going on, but focus on telling your story as if you were speaking with a relative or a friend.

✚ *If there is a diagnosis that you are particularly concerned about, let your doctor know up front.* The doctor may be trying to "rule out" a breast infection, but if you're worried about breast cancer, you may not get the answers you're looking for. If you are concerned about seeming too presumptuous, you can always say something like, "Look, I'm not a doctor or anything, but I have a cousin who had these same symptoms and she ended up being diagnosed with breast cancer. Should I be worried?" Sharing your fears can help your doctor consider a wider list of possibilities, and also make sense that your concerns are addressed.

✚ *Write it down.* Your story may be long and winding, with twists and turns that aren't necessarily straightforward. To help make sure the important parts of the story aren't left out, you can ✚ *use our worksheets* and write down your story. The next time you are going to the doctor, complete the worksheet before you go (or take it with you and complete it in the waiting room). For most situations, we advise you to start with the basic worksheet. If your story is very involved or if you have a particularly complicated set of symptoms, you can use the more in-depth version.

If you are experiencing symptoms over days to weeks, it might help to ✚ *keep a journal.* You can also use the journal to keep track of other aspects of your daily life (activities, eating habits, sleep patterns, times you take medications, and so on) to the extent that you think they may relate to your symptoms. This information can be incredibly helpful in leading you and your doctor to your diagnosis and, later, in tracking your response to treatment.

"What about my past medical history—how much of that should I go into?"

✚ *Carry a card.* It's helpful if you can provide a bullet-point summary of your past medical history so that your doctor can spend more time with you listening to your story. We advise that everyone carry a card in their wallets listing their medical and surgical history, medications, allergies, as well as emergency contact numbers (including your doctor's and next-of-kin contact information). There are several Web sites that will make these cards for you for free. For example, MedId.com has a template that you can input your information into, and within a matter of minutes, a wallet-sized card is generated.[2] Here is a screenshot of a card that we made within two minutes for sample patient "Jane Smith":

⊕ **EMERGENCY MEDICAL IDENTIFICATION**
Courtesy of MedIDs.com

Jane A. Smith DOB: 01/01/1951
commonwealth
Boston, MA 02116 jane.a.smith@~~gmail.com~~
617-222-3▓▓▓ - 617-111-2▓▓▓ Blood Type: A+
Insurance: Blue Cross Blue Shields #:0001-
2222-3333-4444

Emergency Contacts:
Joe Smith-husband-617-222-▓▓▓ -
847-111-▓▓▓
Jenny Smith - daughter - 617-23▓▓▓-

Physicians:
John Martin - 617-123▓▓▓
Alan Gold - 617-234▓▓▓
Mass General Hospital

Conditions/History:
atrial fibrillation, hypertension, depression,
high cholesterol

Medications:
coumadin 1mg every night - hydrochlorothia-
zide 12.5mg once a day - lipitor 40mg every
night - asprin 81mg once a day - effexor 25mg
once a day

Allergies/Other:
Penicillin: lip swelling sulfa drugs: itching
Card Printed: 8/26/2011
Courtesy of MedIDs.com©

Cut around outer edge of above card; fold in half; laminate for durability
Current card size (folded in half: 3.5 x 2 inches

No matter what your past medical history contains, ✚ *remember to include these three most important items when telling your story to the doctor.* First, *mention if there have been any recent changes in your medical history.* Bring up any new developments, however tangential they may seem to the issue at hand. Were you recently hospitalized? Did you just have an operation? Were you in a car accident? Second, ✚ *tell the doctor about any new medications or dosing adjustments.* Include over-the-counter and herbal supplements, as well as prescription medications. If you've started or stopped something, whether on the advice of a doctor or on your own accord, explain why. Third, ✚ *talk about any important changes in your lifestyle or living situation.* Have there been changes to your consumption of alcohol, smoking, or drugs? Do you have a new job, a recent divorce, or a change in your living situation—did your mother-in-law just move in with your family? Are there any other specific life stressors? These questions are also on the worksheets provided. Such details provide the social context that not only bring your story to life, but also allows you and your doctor to develop a more comprehensive understanding of your diagnosis.

Pillar #2: Assert yourself in the doctor's thought process

"The doctor finished asking me for my story and then stuck a stethoscope on my chest. I know I'm supposed to ask to get involved, but I can't stop the physical exam once it's started!"

Sure you can. It's your body and your health. You can say, very nicely, "Excuse me, doctor, I'm sorry to interrupt, but I was just wondering what it is we are looking for? Can you tell me what you're thinking so far after listening to my story?"

"But my doctor is still not telling me anything. She says she doesn't know yet."

The doctor must know something. She must have some inclination. If she doesn't, she should. So ✚ **ask the doctor again.** "After hearing my story, what do you think this might be?"

If she proceeds to examine you without giving you an answer, ✚ **try a slightly different tactic.** "You said you weren't sure, but can you tell me some of the possibilities you are considering?" If your doctor still seems puzzled, ask what you can do for help. For example, "Is there anything else I can offer about my history that would help you narrow down some of the possibilities?"

"She says that before we get to any discussion, we need to do a 'workup' for this and a 'rule-out' for that."

✚ **Play dumb.** You know all about "workups" and "rule-outs" because you're reading this book. But you're not interested in "doctor talk;" you just want help figuring out what your symptoms mean. You want to get to your diagnosis. Continue to ask the questions that you need answered, like: "What's your leading diagnosis at this point?"

If she persists in this line of thinking, ✚ **ask what it is she is "working up".** She should at least offer you a few different diagnoses that she is thinking about. Otherwise why is she doing the "work up" at all?

Your doctor may not be prepared for this line of questioning, so you may want to wade gently into this territory. At the same time, ✚ **don't be too afraid of offending your doctor.** You are an equal partner in your own healthcare, and you are entitled to advocate for yourself. Doctors are used to being challenged throughout their training. You shouldn't be afraid to challenge them in matters that affect your life. Just make sure you do so in a polite and respectful manner, and to always treat your doctor with the same courtesy as how you would want to be treated.

"Doctors always seem to be in a hurry. What happens if my doctor is impatient and doesn't answer my questions—or resists my efforts to share in my physical exam or their thought process?"

First and foremost, if you have a choice of doctors, **+ go to a doctor who welcomes your active participation in your diagnostic process**. Choose someone who makes time to listen to you and answer your questions, who encourages your participation in their thought process, and who engages you in a discussion of your diagnosis. By the same token, watch out for doctors who display signs of impatience, intolerance, condescension, or inflexibility—most likely, these doctors may be relying on cookbook medicine to compensate for their lack of comfort with real people and their stories.

Many times, though, you do not have a choice of doctors. You are stuck with the resident who sees you in the ER or the cardiologist taking care of your ailing mother in the cardiac unit, or there may only be one cancer specialist or family doctor that your insurance allows you to see. Don't despair! In most cases, you *can* make a difference and change how your doctor approaches your care. The vast majority of doctors who practice cookbook medicine actually mean well; they're just used to doing things a certain way. They need help—your help—to see how they can do it differently.

Some suggestions for when you encounter a cookbook doctor:

+ Allow your doctor to get to know you. Tell the doctor a bit about yourself and let him start to feel comfortable with you as his patient. Try not to be threatening at the outset. Don't question his credentials or challenge his approach right off the bat. The last thing you want is a cookbook doctor—or any doctor—who is feeling defensive.

+ Set the expectation that you want a partnership approach to your healthcare. Ask to be involved in the narrative, the physical exam, the differential diagnosis, the decision-making process, and so forth. Make it clear up front that you are willing to accept shared responsibility.

✦ *Ensure that you are listened to.* If your story is interrupted by close-ended questions, insist on telling your story. If your doctor begins to look at her watch and show other signs of impatience (or, as has happened, frankly tells you that she is too busy), look her in the eye and say, politely, "Excuse me, doctor, but I am not finished. May I go on and tell you about what brings me here today?"

✦ *Tell a coherent story.* The more sense you make, the more understandable and clear the story is, the more the doctor will hear you out. Use the tips above to tell a tight and coherent story. Thinking through it beforehand and writing down key elements on the worksheet will help to focus you. If you tell a good story, you give no reason for the doctor *not* to listen to you.

✦ *Ask questions.* If something doesn't make sense, speak up immediately. You shouldn't let these moments pass by anyway, but especially with an impatient doctor, stop them when you have the chance. Even cookbook doctors see value in educating patients, and you can use this to your advantage. Ask about any diagnosis that comes up. Ask why the "workup" should apply to you. Ask if everyone with your symptoms really needs the "rule-out." Give the doctor any opportunity to refocus their attention on your story and your partnership with them.

✦ *Practice all the Pillars.* Your doctor may be in a hurry, but you're not, and you are the one who will be affected the most. Don't skip steps because you feel sorry for your doctor: it's your health at stake here, not theirs, and your doctor is there to help you. Don't give in to someone else's time pressure at the expense of your own health.

✦ *Insist on the care you deserve.* Sometimes you just have to be more assertive (but always, in a courteous and respectful manner). If your doctor says he's too busy to answer a question or explain a physical exam finding, ask how he will get to your right diagnosis if he is not listening to you and helping you. If your symptom is not urgent, another method to try is to ask if there is a better time to see him—perhaps you can come back when he has more time for you. If your symptom is urgent and you are getting nowhere, ask politely if there may be another doctor who may have more time that day. Your doctor should get the message, and as long as you approach it courteously, he should respond in kind, and start providing you with the care that you deserve. Who knows, perhaps this could be the turning point for your doctor to practice differently with future patients, too.

If all of these strategies fail, your last resort is to ✚ *see another doctor as quickly as possible*. Perhaps your ER doctor isn't being helpful—try to follow up with your primary care doctor the next morning. You can even call the on-call doctor for your primary care doctor and speak to them while you're still in the ER. Perhaps the resident taking care of you is in a rush or is having a bad day—ask to see the attending (perhaps even ask the resident to page the attending for you). Perhaps the specialist your primary doctor referred you to doesn't answer your questions—call your primary care doctor for clarification, or ask for another referral. Doctors are here to serve patients, and you can help them become better doctors, for you and for their other patients.

Pillar #3: Participate in your physical exam

"I didn't go to medical school. How can I know what part of the physical exam the doctor is supposed to do?"

This is one reason to ✚ *have the conversation before the physical exam*. Ask about your differential diagnosis and what things your doctor is looking for on the exam. That way, you will know what to expect during the physical exam, and you can add to it elements that you think might be important to be checked out. It also makes it easier to ask the doctor what she has found and what that means.

"So how I can make sure that the doctor is getting the most out of my exam?"

If you have a specific complaint, ✚ *expose that part of your body*. Your knee hurts—take off your pants and make sure the doctor can see clearly your knee, if not your entire leg. If you feel generally unwell and there is not one clear body part that is the problem, ✚ *undress into the gown provided to you*. Help make it easier to examine your whole body. This is particularly important if you are assisting an elderly parent or a child. Being willing to undress also signifies your willingness to participate in the physical exam process, and sends a strong signal that you are going to be a partner in diagnosis.

✦ *Describe your symptoms as specifically as you can during the physical exam.* If you have abdominal pain, point to the location and describe what it feels like when the doctor palpates that area. If you have a rash, describe how it spread, and make sure the entire area is exposed for the doctor to see. This is one more opportunity to tell your story if you feel that the doctor hasn't heard it well enough before.

✦ *Make sure you point out anything unusual or anything you are concerned about.* Something seemingly unrelated—like bruising or swollen glands—may actually be very relevant. Point these things out as the doctor is doing the physical exam.

"Won't the doctor be offended that I'm telling him how to do his job?"

But you're not. You're simply pointing out, on your body, the things that are concerning to you. You are simply partnering with your doctor to make sure that no physical exam clues are missed that may be central to making the diagnosis.

Pillar #4: Make the differential diagnosis together

"My doctor hasn't told me what she's thinking."

✦ *If you want to know what your doctor is thinking, ask her!* You're not a mind reader, and neither is she. You may have to ask a lot of questions to get started, so pick one question to start with, and if it doesn't work, use another one: "What kind of conditions do you think could be causing my symptoms? Would that diagnosis cause me to feel this way? What are some other symptoms that patients with this diagnosis typically experience? How does this diagnosis tie together the other symptoms I have? Can we go through my differential diagnosis? Could I have an unusual presentation of something more common? What less common diagnoses should we be thinking of?" The key is to assert yourself in the diagnostic process as early on as possible.

If you still do not feel like you are getting anywhere, try the following approach. Say, "I know what it is I'm worried about. Can you explain to me what it is you are worried about?" This might be a good entry point for formulating a list that will develop into your differential diagnosis.

"I don't understand the list of things that the doctor came up with for the differential diagnosis."

If the differential diagnosis doesn't make sense to you, it's unlikely you'll be happy with your working diagnosis or treatment plan. Why not get it right from the start? **✦ If you have a problem with the differential diagnosis, speak up and ask for clarification.** Is there a diagnosis that you don't really understand or a diagnosis that doesn't seem to account for your symptoms? Ask about it. Does your doctor's concern about a particular diagnosis seem excessive? Let your doctor know. Is it because there is another diagnosis you are more worried about? Express your concern. Don't be shy to offer alternate possibilities or to ask your doctor to think through the differential again with you.

Pillar #5: Partner for the decision-making process

"My doctor never explained what tests he ordered and why. He just had the nurse come in and draw my blood. What should I do the next time this happens?"

✦ Ask to speak to the doctor again. Doctors should be communicating the plan with their patients prior to it being implemented by other members of staff. Ask your nurse to please find the doctor because you have some questions about your care.

Then, when the doctor arrives, inquire politely, "Doctor, I want to clarify what tests are being done and why. How will these tests bring us closer to a diagnosis? Will the results change what we're planning to do? Do we expect them to be helpful in some other way?"

If all else fails, **✦ flatter the doctor.** As the patient, you can't be expected to know everything! Let the doctor be the expert. It's the doctor's job to explain what the alternatives are when it comes to testing—what a particular test is meant to show, or not show; how likely it is that a given test is going to inform the differential diagnosis in your particular case; etc. Say to the doctor, "Doctor, you are the expert on these conditions. Would you mind to please explain the test to me, just so that I can understand?"

"I understand that there are lots of tests out there, but how can I be expected to know which ones make sense?"

Before a decision can be discussed at all, the doctor has to give you a working diagnosis, or at least a list of possible diagnoses: the differential diagnosis. ✚ *If you get the sense that your doctor is ordering tests without any thought about the differential diagnosis, you need to start over.* Ask you doctor if he would mind going over what he thinks you have. "Can we go through what it is I might have, and then talk about how these tests can help narrow that list down?"

"My doctor said I need more tests because we don't want to miss 'something serious.' How scared should I be?"

As we discussed, any symptom from chest pain to a scraped knee *could* be serious. The question is not whether it's theoretically possible, but how likely it is to be the case. ✚ *If your doctor is saying you need more tests, ask why.* What diagnosis is he afraid of missing? How likely does she think it is, and what would be the consequences of missing it? And what is the diagnosis she thinks you have—and how likely is that diagnosis, as compared to other diagnoses (both life-threatening or not)? You have to have some knowledge of probabilities if you are to make any decisions about what to do next.

If the doctor isn't able to give you probabilities, try a different approach. ✚ *Ask your doctor what he would do if he were the patient, or his family member were the patient.* You may have a different risk tolerance from your doctor, and he may make different decisions than you would, but hearing about what the doctor would do for himself or a loved one gives you a sense of how urgent he perceives your condition to be. If your doctor says that he would absolutely encourage his wife to get the same tests if she were in the same position, that would likely also change your outlook on the severity of your condition. On the other hand, if the doctor would not recommend for his loved one to be hospitalized, it would help confirm your inclination—and also help the doctor see your point of view.

Pillar #6: Apply tests rationally

"The doctor quoted a bunch of statistics, but I'm not sure I really understand why I have to do this test."

✦ **If the doctor isn't answering your questions in a way that makes sense to you, rephrase the question.** Try asking other related questions that also get to the heart of the matter. "Can you explain again the pros/cons of doing this test?" might be one approach. "Are there any alternatives to this test?" would be another way to ask. You need to agree with the diagnostic approach that is being used on you, and you should walk away from the doctor's visit feeling listened to, understood, and empowered—in general, feeling good about the discussion.

"The result of the first test is back, and the doctor is saying that I need to get more tests done. What should I be asking?"

To begin with, ✦ **you should know what the test was looking for.** What was the purpose of that test in the first place? How relevant are the results to your condition? If the purpose was to check if you have pancreatitis, and a test looking for this is abnormal, then perhaps a further test is reasonable. On the other hand, if the purpose was looking for pancreatitis, but a separate abnormal result—say, an elevated white blood cell count—was obtained, you might question the importance of this finding. We discussed how many results are "incidental" findings, because the range of what is normal is quite wide. ✦ **Ask your doctor what any abnormal result means.** White blood cell counts, for example, are elevated in so many conditions as to be quite meaningless a lot of the time. Make sure you understand the significance of a "positive" or "abnormal" result.

If a new series of tests is now being suggested based on the first abnormal result, ✦ **ask what you will learn from doing this second round of testing.** Is this yet another "rule-out," or is this going to provide a definitive answer? And if this is another rule-out, where does it stop?

Sometimes, it may not be necessary to do the test to get that definitive answer. Patients who have diarrhea rarely need stool cultures to find out exactly what kind of virus is causing their symptoms—it's fine to begin treatment. ✦ **Ask if it's necessary to do the test to confirm a working diagnosis.** Is it even necessary to get to a definitive diagnosis?

"Honestly, I'm still lost. Is there anything else I can do to express my concern about the test to my doctor?"

One of our colleagues at the Brigham and Women's, Dr. Ali Raja, provides the following advice: ✚ *talk to the nurses.* Many times, it is nurses who spend more of their time with their patients and have both the time to hear the patients' concerns and also the authority to address them with their doctors.

If you have trouble getting through to your doctor, Dr. Raja recommends that you say to your nurse, "I feel like something is wrong. I haven't gotten all the information I wanted from the doctor. Can you or she explain more?"

This is excellent advice. Nurses can help you advocate for your health, so enlist their help if you feel like you are having trouble getting through to your doctor, about a test, or about other aspects of your care.

Pillar #7: Use common sense to confirm the working diagnosis

"The doctor gave me a working diagnosis, but I'm pretty sure he's off base. I don't want to seem rude, though."

✚ *There are ways to question your diagnosis without having to challenge your doctor's judgment.* Say the doctor thinks you have acid reflux, but you're still worried about your heart. Point out (respectfully) why it is that you are concerned. "Doctor, if this is really just acid reflux, why did it start all of a sudden? I've never had problems with heartburn before?" or "How does heartburn explain the pressure I feel in my chest when I climb the stairs?" ✚ *Remember the power of the "why" and "how" questions.* If your doctor isn't asking them, you should be.

Another approach is to ✚ *ask what else could explain your symptoms and how the doctor is sure you don't have these things.* Perhaps the doctor has a solid rationale, in which case you may be reassured by her response. If she doesn't, perhaps she would be prompted to by your questions.

If what you are saying still fails to get her attention, ✚ *be direct with your doctor.* "I am afraid that we are missing something here. From the little I know of this diagnosis, it doesn't seem to fit with my symptoms. Is there anything else that my symptoms could indicate?"

"My doctor mentioned a diagnosis that I had never heard of. I don't know what I don't know. How would I know if it fits or not?"

✦ **Start by asking the doctor to explain what he knows about the diagnosis.** Does it fit with what your symptoms are? Take the opportunity while you have your doctor's attention to ask questions. Ask your nurse, and ask to see your doctor again if you need to get further clarification.

✦ *Do your own research.* In today's day and age, you can do this practically wherever you find yourself—whether at home, in the doctor's office, or in the ER. Google the diagnosis on your smartphone. Call a friend or family member who might know, or who can look it up for you. Learn what you can about the diagnosis, but most important, find out what questions you should be asking your doctor.

✦ *Be particularly wary if the doctor seems focused on one particular diagnosis* and is using a cookbook recipe to "rule it out" or "work it up." Question whether you were being put on one particular pathway to look for just one problem. Always ask, what *else* can this be?

✦ *Look out for cookbook mentality.* Even when the doctor isn't following a specific recipe, he may still be using cookbook thinking that is subject to all the pitfalls we've seen. Be open with your doctor about it, and ask questions. "What pathway are you following to figure out whether I have this? What tests are you ordering, and what happens if they don't lead us to a diagnosis? Can we work together to come up with a differential diagnosis? What *else* do you think I would have? Can we make a list together of the differential diagnosis?" and so forth.

"The doctor told me I'm fine, but he never really told me what was wrong in the first place? Is it OK to leave without a diagnosis?"

By now, you know that the answer is a resounding *no.* ✦ *Do not leave your doctor's office without at least a working diagnosis.* Without some idea of what is going on with you, how can the doctor be sure that you are going to be OK? What if she's wrong? How will you know what to expect going forward? Again, without being aggressive, it's perfectly find to ask, "So, at the end of the day, what do you think was causing my symptoms? What do you think it could have been?"

"The diagnosis passed my reality check, but now I've done more research on it and it doesn't seem to fit. What now?"

✚ *It's always important that you have a clear follow-up plan.* Were you supposed to follow a treatment and then see the same doctor for a repeat appointment? Were you supposed to see a primary care doctor or a specialist for follow-up? If your concerns are not urgent, you can address them at this repeat appointment; sometimes, more information can lead to a more accurate diagnosis the second time around. If they are urgent, consider seeing a doctor sooner and perhaps even going to a different doctor to seek a second opinion. When you come for a second visit, ✚ *make sure you revise your worksheet* to include all of the new things that have happened since your last visit.

"I developed new symptoms, but how do I know if they're serious or not?"

✚ *Before the doctor leaves, make sure he tells you what to expect.* You should make sure that you received instructions about the natural history of whatever diagnosis the doctor suspects: the expected time course for your symptoms to resolve (with or without treatment), additional symptoms you might experience, and what other symptoms you should *not* have. Know when you should follow up and with whom.

✚ *The "red flag" symptoms that the doctor identifies should make sense to you.* If there is any uncertainty about your diagnosis (and there often is), know what signs or symptoms to look out for (the so-called "red flags") that may warn you of a potentially more serious diagnosis. For example, after a neck injury, numbness or tingling in one hand usually means a pinched nerve on one side, which is generally a benign process, whereas numbness in both arms, or weakness, may signify a problem with the spinal cord. Knowing what you are supposed to look out for helps to inform you; you should know not just what you're watching out for but why.

"My doctor couldn't settle on one diagnosis. She thinks my symptoms may be caused by a few different things. Is this OK?"

Yes. Your doctor is giving you several working diagnoses. The key is to ✚ *make sure you understand what differentiates one working diagnosis from the other.* Know what to expect in each case. What is the worst that can happen in each of the cases? What would distinguish one disease from the other? When, if at all, should you come back to further narrow down the diagnosis?

+ *Before you leave your doctor, always ask one last time: is there any-thing* else *that can explain my symptoms*? Perform one final common sense check before you leave. Even if you have two, or more, working diagnoses, make sure there is nothing else that was eliminated as a possibility too soon—or was never considered. Know the warning signs of these dis-eases, too.

Pillar #8: Integrate diagnosis into the healing process

Our book focuses on diagnosis and does not specifically address treat-ment, but there is such a thing as treatment that incorporates the same ele-ments of shared decision-making and active partnership. In order to begin any kind of treatment, there should be a diagnosis. Coming up with a diag-nosis is the first step to understanding symptoms and to feeling better. This is an intuitive part of every patient's understanding. Here are some sugges-tions for moving forward, once you have a working diagnosis.

"I asked about what to expect in my illness, and my doctor shrugged and said she doesn't know, that everyone's different. How can I get her to tell me more?"

Understanding the expected course of your illness is a necessary com-ponent on the journey to getting better. Your doctor should be willing to share this with you. Perhaps she is uncomfortable predicting because she is not sure herself, and doesn't want to tell you unless she is absolutely sure. + *Assure your doctor that you don't need her to be 100 percent certain, but that you want to know what she knows.* Say that you realize she may not know how exactly your illness will evolve, but what is typical for patients with this diagnosis? What has been her experience with other patients? Sometimes, doctors don't tell patients what to expect because they don't think that patients can handle uncertainty. But what they don't realize is that being told nothing brings about even more uncertainty than an honest, open discussion. It's true that every patient is different: some may recover faster on their own, some may respond better to one treat-ment over another. Adding to this uncertainty, it's quite possible that, at the end of the day, after all the thinking and tests, your doctor is still not entirely sure what you have. But this, too, is information you should know, and you should let your doctor feel comfortable sharing these nuances with you.

"My doctor admitted to me that he honestly did not know much about this illness. He recommended that I see a specialist. But I can't get an appointment to see this person for weeks. What should I do?"

Your doctor presumably knows *something* about the diagnosis. Even if he is not an expert in that field, he should at least know where to look up information about it. While it's good that your doctor recognizes his limitations, he should at least be able to answer for you some basic questions, such as: why you think I have this illness? What is the natural course of this illness? What's the worst thing that can happen? What are some steps I can take to feel better, while I'm waiting to see a specialist? If he doesn't bring these topics up himself, you should ask. ✦ *If your doctor says he doesn't know, ask him if he can find out and get back to you.*

"When I asked my doctor about treatment, he made it sound like there was just one treatment available. I feel like I have no options."

✦ *There are always choices available to you.* You should think hard about a doctor who is trying to convince you that there is only one right way. Many aspects of medicine lack clear-cut, right-or-wrong answers. There may be situations that require a very specific intervention, but in most cases, there are reasonable alternatives. Everything has a trade-off, whether it's side effects of medications or a risk of a procedure. Your doctor should be willing to talk through these with you. If you are presented with only one option, ask about alternatives.

✦ *If you are still hearing only one option, ask the question in a different way.* "What happens if I do nothing?" or "What happens if I postpone the decision?" There are some rare emergencies that require a very specific intervention (for example, flesh-eating bacteria that requires immediate surgery), but in almost all cases, there are alternatives. Before you can weigh the risks and benefits of these, you need to hear all of your options, and your doctor needs to tell you.

"I agree with all of this! But how can I choose a doctor who practices medicine in the way that you propose? And what happens if I don't have a choice?"

A good doctor is someone who cares about you as an individual. She should see medical practice as a lifelong learning process, and be willing to refine her practice with each patient, striving to get better rather than to stagnate in cookbook patterns. She should be a good communicator. She should welcome your inquiries and be comfortable answering all your questions. She should listen to your story, and actively involve you in every step of the diagnostic and decision-making process. She should prioritize your diagnosis and make sure that you are provided one by the end of your visit.

This is the ideal doctor who will guide you through the process of making your correct diagnosis and lead you to the right treatment. This doctor, though, is few and far in between, and most of us will not have the choice of selecting her. Or perhaps we have a choice, but can't tell what doctor will be closest to this ideal presented.

If you do have a choice of doctors, that's great. You can decide, based on your interactions, whether he or she will be open to a partnership approach toward finding your diagnosis. If you don't, then this is your chance to teach them how medical care can and should be. Incorporate the principles we've talked about and advocate for the best care for yourself. Doctors may be practicing cookbook medicine out of habit, or may feel compelled to do so because it's become such standard practice and it's what they think their patients expect. Show them that your expectations are different. Demonstrate how a patient-centered approach that emphasizes diagnosis can work **+** *Make your doctor into the ideal doctor that you always wanted by showing them the way!*

Mrs. Ware is doing well. We know this because Jessica is our literary agent, the one who recognized and believed in the value in our approach to medical care from the start. Having read a draft of our book by the time this incident occurred, she was well aware of the key role of the narrative and the importance of partnering in the diagnostic process.

"My friend was probably just dehydrated after all," Jessica tells us. "But we were scared. Now, I know firsthand how disorienting it can be when you're being bombarded by all of these questions, while none of *your* questions are being answered. Patients and those with them need guidance in these vulnerable moments."

This is all the more reason to use the worksheets, understand the 8 Pillars, and prepare ahead of time through these Prescriptions for Patients. We urge you to read through this chapter again. As you go through it this time, take a look at Appendix 2. Read through the corresponding exercises that you can practice today—before you have any need to go see your doctor. Being ill, or watching your loved one suffer, is disorientating and frightening, but you can prepare yourself so that you get the right diagnosis and the right care.

911 REVIEW

- If you have a choice of doctors, select one who engages you as an equal partner in the diagnostic process.
- You may not have a choice of doctors. There are still many things you can to do make sure that your doctor practices the type of medicine you deserve.
- Practice the Prescriptions for Patients and the 8 Pillars today.
- Never be afraid to speak up. It's your health; you need to advocate for it.

Fifteen

Cookbook Outcomes, Revisited

In this chapter, we revisit the four cases from Part II. Instead of the cookbook approach that was used the first time around, we will see how these same patients can become active participants in their diagnosis to achieve vastly different outcomes. Of course, the actual patients in these four cases were not able to reenact these scenarios, but we attempt to use their voice to demonstrate how ordinary people like them, like all of us, can lead the way to avoiding misdiagnosis. Take note of their style and technique in applying the 8 Pillars to Better Diagnosis. Focus on the ✚ 911 Action Tips that we use to highlight particularly effective dialogue; these should look familiar to you from the last chapter's Prescriptions for Patients. Think about what you would do if you were in their shoes: can you advocate for your care as they did? What will you need to work on in order to do that?

Jerry, the Car Mechanic with the Pulled Muscle

Remember Jerry, the forty-eight-year-old who developed chest pain after helping his brother move? He arrived at the ER and was promptly labeled with a chief complaint of "chest pain" and got a battery of tests done as part of the "chest pain pathway." These tests continued throughout the night and into the next day, when he finally was allowed to leave, but without any real diagnosis.

Let's turn back the clock. Jerry has gone through triage and had his EKG. He's been waiting anxiously to see the doctor. We catch up with him as the doctor enters his room:

DOCTOR: So what brings you here today?

JERRY: Well, I was helping my brother move his things to a new place over the weekend. Today, I woke up with this kinda tight pain in my chest. I think it's just a pulled muscle, but my wife, she got scared and thought maybe it's a heart attack—

DOCTOR: When did the chest pain start?

JERRY: I guess I woke up with it. It's not a pain, more of a soreness. It got worse when I moved around and it hurts when I touch my chest.

DOCTOR: Does it radiate anywhere?

JERRY: No, it just stayed in my chest, on both sides. Like I said, it's not always there. I notice it most when I move around.

DOCTOR: Do you have trouble breathing? Any nausea? Vomiting?

JERRY: No, none of that. Do you think it's related to my moving all that heavy furniture? Like I pushed myself too hard or something?

DOCTOR: It could be, but chest pain is something to be taken seriously. It could be a heart attack.

JERRY: Do you really think it could be a heart attack?

DOCTOR: Well, for our patients with chest pain, especially at your age, we have to think about life-threatening problems like a heart attack. Sure, it could be a muscle pull, too, but we always want to be on the safe side and "rule out" the worst-case scenarios.

JERRY: Sure. I get that. And you would know better than me about the type

---

✚ 911 ACTION TIP

If your doctor keeps on asking you close-ended questions, answer them, but then ask him questions back. Attach narrative responses to his close-ended questions.

✚ 911 ACTION TIP

Early on, make it clear that you expect to be a partner in the diagnostic process.

---

of things that would point to one diagnosis or another. Would you mind explaining them to me as we go along?

DOCTOR: Sure. So far, nothing that I've heard so far is terribly concerning. [He gestures to Jerry to sit up as he pulls out his stethoscope.] Any family history of heart problems? Anything like this happen before?

JERRY: No, no. . . . Doctor, while you're doing the physical exam, can you point out what you're looking for?

DOCTOR: [listens to heart and lungs, then presses on chest] Sure, I can try.

JERRY: Right there, doctor, where your stethoscope is . . . a little to the right . . . that's where it hurts the most.

DOCTOR: How about this, does this hurt when I press?

JERRY: [wincing] Wow, that really smarts. See, that's why I thought it was a muscle pull. It also hurts when I twist like this from side to side.

DOCTOR: Yes, that would be consistent with a muscle strain. Still, . . .

JERRY: How were my heart and lungs?

DOCTOR: I didn't hear a murmur in your heart. Your lungs sounded clear. So now, we wait for your labs to come back. We should also get an X-ray of your chest.

JERRY: So are we still thinking I could have a heart attack?

DOCTOR: Umm, no, not really. But I'd like to run some tests just to be sure.

JERRY: Do you think it's necessary to do more tests at this point? Or is there something else we should be worried about?

✚ 911 ACTION TIP

Describe symptoms as specifically as you can during the physical exam. Point out anything unusual and what you are concerned about.

DOCTOR: Well, I think you probably have a pulled muscle. It's very unlikely you have a collapsed lung or a clot in your lungs that's causing you this pain. I don't think you broke a rib.

JERRY: So it's probably a pulled muscle, right? So how come we have to do tests?

DOCTOR: Well, we have something called the "chest pain pathway" for our patients who come in with chest pain.

JERRY: OK, but maybe I'm not like every other patient with chest pain. What about the "Jerry" pathway?

DOCTOR: I guess so. . . . Listen, we have the pathway so we can save time for you. And I need to run. So you'll get some tests done now, OK?

JERRY: Actually, doctor, I'm not OK with that. It doesn't sound like it's going to save me time to do tests that I don't need. I know you are busy, but I also want to know what's the plan here. Can you explain again to me the tests that are being done and what they're supposed to show? Or if you're busy now, perhaps we can talk when you have a minute to spare?

DOCTOR: [sighs] OK. You've had your EKG and it looked normal. You already got blood drawn so we can wait for that to come back. We would normally keep someone like you here overnight. I think we should, to be on the safe side, and do what we call a stress test in the morning.

JERRY: So let me see if I understand. The EKG was normal—I assume that's good news. I already got blood drawn so sure, we can wait for that. If that's all OK, why would I have to stay overnight?

DOCTOR: Because sometimes EKGs and blood tests don't show damage to your heart immediately. It's important that you stay overnight and complete more blood tests in the morning. And we can do a stress test for you, which is when you run on the treadmill and we see whether that causes strain on your heart.

✚ 911 ACTION TIP

If your doctor says something that doesn't make sense, ask for clarification. If you don't agree with the plan, let her know right away.

JERRY: But you were just saying that it's very unlikely I'm having a heart at-tack. Like less than 5 percent? [Doctor nods.] And if all the blood tests come back normal, then the chance is even lower, would you say less than 1 percent? [Doctor nods.] I mean, you know much more than I do about the value of tests. Can you help me understand how it would help to go through these extra tests?

DOCTOR: I suppose they don't add that much. It's just to be extra-safe. I do think you probably have a pulled muscle and that explains all your symptoms.

JERRY: If you were me, what would you do? Would you stay in the hospital for extra tests?

DOCTOR: No, because I'd be pretty sure I just had a muscle strain. You make a good point. OK, why don't we do this? If your labs look fine, you can go home, as long as you promise to come back if your pain gets worse.

JERRY: Worse? I want it to get better!

DOCTOR: Of course. Well, if it's a muscle strain, like we think it is, it should get better with time. Some rest and some ibuprofen should get you feel-ing better in a day or two.

JERRY: That sounds great. Last question: on the off chance that we did miss something, you know the less than 1 percent chance we talked about, what should I be on the lookout for?

DOCTOR: Well, like I said, a muscle strain should only last for a couple of days, and it should pretty much stay in the same place. You really shouldn't

---

✚ 911 ACTION TIP

To get a better sense of risk, ask the doctor what he would do if he or his family member were the patient.

✚ 911 ACTION TIP

Always make sure you know what to do to make yourself feel better. Know what to expect, including the bad things that may happen if the di-agnosis is wrong.

develop any new symptoms (aside from, perhaps, a bit of stomach upset if you're sensitive to the ibuprofen). If you start to have worsening pain, or any other new symptoms, I would be concerned that something else may be going on.

JERRY: Doc, thanks for taking the time to explain everything to me and for involving me in the decision-making process. That's really helpful.

DOCTOR: You're welcome. I'll write up your discharge instructions.

How different is this version of the story from the one that happened, when Jerry ended up waiting all night for a stress test he couldn't complete, then got discharged with a huge bill but didn't actually feel any better? This new version is the one that Jerry himself wishes he could have had.

In this version, Jerry followed the 8 Pillars to Better Diagnosis. From the start, he insisted on telling his whole story (#1). He fought the attempt to pigeonhole his symptoms as "chest pain" and countered the many dichotomous questions with explanations rather than yes/no answers. Even before the physical exam, he asserted his own narrative and expressed his concerns (#2). He was an active participant in his own physical exam, pointing out what hurt him and leading the doctor to see how this corresponded to the diagnosis of muscle strain (#3). In so doing, he also learned that he had a normal heart and lung exam, something that he could remember for the future.

Then, Jerry asked about the differential diagnosis (#4) and challenged the assumption that he belonged in a "chest pain pathway" and the worst-case reasoning that came with the recipe (#5). He insisted on remaining an integral part of the decision-making process, and when the doctor expressed impatience with him, he found a polite but firm way to state his point. As a partner in the diagnostic process, he pointed out what he thought made sense and what didn't and asked for the rationale behind tests (#6). He helped his doctor understand his own decision-making process, and ensured that they arrived together at a good working diagnosis (#7) with an understanding of his likely prognosis and an appropriate treatment plan (#8).

Annette, the Mother of Two Who Had Trouble Breathing

Annette Golding was our thirty-two-year-old overweight woman who had gotten progressively more tired and more out of breath. It turned out that her symptoms were consistent with a diagnosis of obstructive sleep apnea all along. Yet, it took doctors many weeks and mountains unnecessary and invasive to make the diagnosis. In fact, it all started because her primary care doctor was concerned that she needed to be "ruled out" for a pulmonary embolism and sent her to the ER.

Let's see what happens this time, when Annette shows up to the ER with the slip of paper from her primary care doctor that read: "Obese smoker, birth control pills, recent plane trip, persistent SOB—rule out PE."

DOCTOR: Good evening, Mrs. Golding. I see that your primary care doctor sent you here because he was concerned about you might have a blood clot in your lungs. How has your breathing been?

ANNETTE: Well, I've been getting more winded recently, but I think it has to do with my overall fatigue—

DOCTOR: Have you had trouble catching your breath?

ANNETTE: Well, a little, but—

DOCTOR: Have you had any chest pain? Any fevers? Chills?

ANNETTE: Not really. The main thing is that I've been getting so tired, for months really. And also winded—like climbing steps or running to catch the bus. I know I'm out of shape, I've gained some weight over the past few years. But it's like I'm tired all the time now. Then I went to Toronto to see my sister and her baby, and when I got back, I just had zero energy.

DOCTOR: What about your shortness of breath? How long has that been going on for?

✚ 911 ACTION TIP

Provide your doctor with context.

ANNETTE: It's been months—mostly climbing stairs and things. My doctor thought it might be my asthma.

DOCTOR: Have you had asthma before?

ANNETTE: Yeah, when I was younger. But I wasn't really wheezing or anything. Though . . . Come to think of it, I did have some other breathing issues recently. My mouth has been dry. And this is kind of embarrassing. I never thought I snored, but my sister and her husband said I snored a lot in my sleep.

DOCTOR: Hmm, that's strange, but that's not really that concerning; right now, I'm worried you may have a clot in your lungs.

ANNETTE: That sounds really serious. Is that why I'm so tired all the time? I mean, I went to see my doctor today because I almost fell asleep when I was driving. My kids were in the car with me. It's never ever happened to me before. I can't let it happen again.

DOCTOR: Well, I'm not sure the blood clot would explain your fatigue, but a pulmonary embolism is a life-threatening diagnosis. We need to do some tests to make sure you don't have it.

ANNETTE: Can I ask you why everyone keeps thinking I have a pulmonary embolism? I'm not even sure I know what one is?

DOCTOR: Umm . . . [checks his watch] Sure. A pulmonary embolism is a clot in the blood vessels of your lungs. It can cause permanent disability and could lead to death. You have a history that's classic for pulmonary em-

---

✚ 911 ACTION TIP

Communicate what's most worrisome to you. This part of the dialogue is also notable for the element of surprise, which you should include to make your story stand out.

✚ 911 ACTION TIP

Correct mistakes as soon as you hear them.

✚ 911 ACTION TIP

Be wary if your doctor seems to focus on one particular disease to "rule out." Ask what else your doctor is thinking. Come up with the differential diagnosis together.

---

bolism. You have shortness of breath after getting off an airplane. You have a history of birth control pill use and smoking.

ANNETTE: But my shortness of breath started a long time before my trip to Toronto. I've got two kids and haven't used birth control pills in years. The last time I smoked was back in college.

DOCTOR: Oh, I didn't know that. Thanks for pointing that out. [makes notes] Still, I'm worried about pulmonary embolism. It's what your primary care doctor sent you here to evaluate. [pager rings]

ANNETTE: Sure, but I want to make sure we considered all the different possibilities. What else do you think this could be? Could it be an infection?

DOCTOR: Nothing about your history really suggests an infection: you don't have a cough, or fever, do you? I don't think it's a heart problem but I'll listen to your heart and lungs and we can do an EKG just to be sure. You haven't started any new medications recently, have you? Benadryl, antihistamines, anything like that? [Annette shakes her head.] So I don't think it's medication-induced, either. Any travel outside of the country, other than to Canada? Or hiking? [Annette shakes her head.] So not likely a parasitic infestation, or Lyme disease. [pager rings again]

ANNETTE: Doctor, I know you're busy. I appreciate your spending the time with me to fully understand my story. Can you think of anything else that might also explain my feeling so tired?

DOCTOR: Sure. There could be things like anemia. Have your periods been heavier than usual? [Annette shakes her head.] Any bleeding in your stools? [No.] Have you been depressed recently? Or feel cold when everyone else feels hot? Any chance you could be pregnant?

ANNETTE: No. Can I ask what you are getting at when you asked those questions?

DOCTOR: [cell phone rings] Um . . . I'm sorry to cut this conversation short,

---

+ 911 ACTION TIP

It is up to you to advocate for the care that you deserve. If the doctor appears too busy for you, gently suggest that you can wait for him to take care of his more pressing issues—that you would like to have a conversation when he is more free.

---

but I'll need to run to see other patients. We can just order your CT scan to make sure you don't have a clot in your lungs, OK?

ANNETTE: Doctor, I know that I am asking you a lot of questions. I see you're busy, but before we order any tests, I'd rather wait for you to come back and spend just a few minutes with me to think through what I might have?

DOCTOR: Sure, sure. [checks his phone] So where were we? We were just thinking through other reasons you could be tired, like anemia, depression, and problems with your thyroid.

ANNETTE: Right. Would any of these relate to the other symptoms I mentioned, like my not sleeping that well at night?

DOCTOR: Well, there is one more thing we can consider. In people who are overweight, there is a higher incidence of obstructive sleep apnea. That's when a person's upper airway closes up during sleep, then when they wake up, they breathe again. The constant sleeping and waking up does make people tired during the day.

ANNETTE: That sounds like me! Do you think I have that?

DOCTOR: It's possible. But I do think we should first make sure you don't have something else more immediately life-threatening, like a pulmonary embolism. We need to do a CT scan.

ANNETTE: Doesn't a CT scan carry a risk of radiation? My mother had Hodgkin's lymphoma from radiation to her thyroid. I don't want anything with that kind of radiation.

DOCTOR: Why don't we do this. There is a blood test we can do that can screen for blood clots and we can use that test to see if we should proceed.

ANNETTE: Let me see if I understand. We have to do this blood test to see if I have a clot in my lungs? And if the blood test is positive, I have to do the CT scan?

✚ 911 ACTION TIP

If you get the sense that your doctor is ordering tests without good reasons, ask questions.

DOCTOR: I think so, yes. We don't want to miss a pulmonary embolism.

ANNETTE: But why are we worried about a pulmonary embolism in the first place? I mean, do patients with pulmonary embolism have stories like mine?

DOCTOR: Well, they do have shortness of breath. They tend to have a faster heart rate and low oxygen saturation. Sometimes they have swelling in their legs.

ANNETTE: I don't have any of that, do I? [Doctor shakes his head] And the history, too. I don't smoke, I haven't used birth control in years, and my travel, that was after my symptoms started.

DOCTOR: You have a point.

ANNETTE: And what about this sleep apnea thing? Is there a test I can do for that?

DOCTOR: All right. You know what? I agree that you're at very low risk for a pulmonary embolism. Here's what we can do. I still think you need a regular chest X-ray to make sure we're not missing a pneumonia. It involves pretty minimal radiation. We can get a blood count to make sure your symptoms aren't due to anemia. And a thyroid test. And I know you told me it's unlikely you're pregnant, but stranger things have happened. If everything checks out, I'll call your primary care doctor and set up for you to get a sleep study. We also need to run this plan by her, too, to be on the safe side. You should be able to go home after that. How does that sound?

ANNETTE: That sounds like a great plan. So what happens if it turns out I have sleep apnea?

✚ 911 ACTION TIP

Ask your doctor what he knows about your working diagnosis.

DOCTOR: You can talk to your primary care doctor more about this, but this is very much a treatable problem. Sometimes people wear masks at night to help them sleep better, for example. For other people, if they lose some weight, the problem goes away.

ANNETTE: Interesting. I don't think I had this problem until I put on all the weight with my last pregnancy.

DOCTOR: There you go!

ANNETTE: Just one more question, doctor—and thank you for bearing with me so far. Is there any long-term damage from this problem?

DOCTOR: There could be. That's why it's important to get it diagnosed early—and why it's good you came to see us for your symptoms.

ANNETTE: I'm definitely glad I did, then. Thank you for hearing me out and coming up with a plan with me.

In this new and improved version, Annette was able to overcome the overwhelming diagnostic momentum that was focused on pulmonary embolism by doing several things. First, she insisted on telling her version of her story from the very start, taking control of the narrative and ensuring that the doctor listened to what she had to say from start to finish (#1). By asking what part of her story was concerning to the doctor, she was able to clarify that she wasn't really a smoker on birth control pills, and that her symptoms hadn't developed suddenly. Note how she steered the doctor in the right direction by emphasizing that the main reason she was seeking care was because her fatigue, and that her shortness of breath had been progressive for months and the other symptoms such as snoring that the doctor hadn't been inclined to take seriously.

Annette continued to drive the narrative by asserting herself in the diagnostic process and asking her doctor for a partnership (#2), particularly when it came to coming up with a differential diagnosis (#4). She brought up several times her concerns with fatigue, and made sure she also mentioned the sleep problems—which turned out to be highly relevant. By challenging the doctor to tie together all the symptoms and her normal physical exam (#3), she got him to think beyond pulmonary embolism and to broaden his differential diagnosis to think about what else she could have (#5). That was how her ultimate diagnosis was reached.

Even so, the doctor had continued to press for tests that she didn't want. Take note of how she was able to express her concerns about radiation associated with the CT scan, and to ask exactly what benefit this test would have in clarifying her diagnosis (#6). She inquired about the alternatives, hoping for something that might make more sense than a cookbook recipe (#7). Take note, too, of how she dealt with her doctor's impatience. Eventually, her doctor came around, and together they agreed on a working diagnosis and a treatment plan (#8).

Danielle, The College Student With a Bad Headache

Remember Danielle? She was the twenty-year-old music student who woke up with a headache after a night on the town with her friends. She was pretty sure she had a bad hangover, and that was what the triage nurse and the resident doctor thought she had, too. Then, the attending heard from a second nurse about her bad headache being the "worst headache of her life", and ordered a head CT and a lumbar puncture (the "subarachnoid pathway") to make sure her headache wasn't something much more serious. When she heard about the plan, Danielle literally ran for it and left the ER without even waiting for her instructions.

Let's revisit her story at the point where she encounters the attending physician.

ATTENDING: Danielle, I'm the supervising doctor in the ER. I heard a bit about your story. It sounds like you're having a pretty bad headache. Did it started suddenly?

DANIELLE: Well, sort of. It started this morning, when I woke up. Actually, I'm not really that sure because I was kind of groggy. I had a late night last night. You know, like with drinking. I normally don't drink very much, maybe one or two beers. Last night I had like two beers and maybe five shots. I think I just crashed when I got home. So the headache was pretty bad when I woke up, but I thought it was because of the drinking.

ATTENDING: Have you had headaches before?

DANIELLE: Yeah, but hasn't everyone? I saw my doctor back home for them.

ATTENDING: Would you say this is the worst headache of your life?

✚ 911 ACTION TIP

Use your own words, as if you were talking to a family member. Stick with simple language rather than medical jargon.

DANIELLE: [pauses] I guess so. My usual headaches are not this bad. The reason I came to the ER, though, was 'cause I felt really light-headed when I tried to get up to go to the bathroom. My friend had to help me sit down 'cause I was getting real woozy. Maybe I was dehydrated. I mean, I wasn't really drinking water all morning, though I tried. Then I threw up and I felt worse.

ATTENDING: You threw up? Just once? [Danielle nods] Are you still nauseous now?

DANIELLE: I feel better now, actually. The IV helped. So maybe what I had was dehydration after all.

ATTENDING: Maybe, but we need to get some tests. [Gathers his paperwork to leave] My resident will come back once all the tests are done.

DANIELLE: Hold on! The other doctor said it's just a hangover. Are you concerned about something else?

ATTENDING: [walks toward door] The resident will explain it to you just now. Take care.

DANIELLE: Doctor, please wait a minute! I'm sorry to bother you about this, because I know you're very busy. You're the one in charge, right? Can I please talk to you about what's going on?

ATTENDING: [sighs] Sure.

DANIELLE: I know you're busy, but can you please help me understand what's going on? The resident didn't seem that concerned, and now you're saying you are—can you please help me understand why?

✚ 911 ACTION TIP

Your doctor should not delegate the patient-physician relationship to someone else. Call him on it—politely.

✚ 911 ACTION TIP

If you identify a discrepancy in what different providers said, clarify as early as you can.

✚ 911 ACTION TIP

Be profuse with your use of "please" and "thank you." Even if you are frustrated and you think the doctor is being rude, remember to remain calm and be courteous.

ATTENDING: Right, well, I'm worried about you. The resident thinks you have a hangover headache, and that might be it. But I think that with such a severe headache, there's a chance you could have a more serious problem. For example, maybe you hit your head last night—

DANIELLE: I didn't!

ATTENDING: You said you were drunk. Maybe it happened without you realizing it.

DANIELLE: But I'm positive I didn't! I never blacked out or anything. My roommates were with me the entire time. Look, if I didn't hit my head, what else could this be?

ATTENDING: You could still have a brain hemorrhage without trauma to your head. You could have meningitis, too. That could also cause a bad headache and vomiting.

DANIELLE: There was an outbreak of meningitis in my sister's dorm when she was a freshman. Wouldn't you be sicker, with fever with that? What else on my physical exam would you be looking for?

ATTENDING: You're right, your story is not particularly good for meningitis, but it *is* a life-threatening issue and always something to consider. Things on physical exam would be a rigid neck, high fever, and certain other signs that my resident already told me you don't have.

DANIELLE: What about a stroke? My mom was worried about me having a stroke.

ATTENDING: Honestly, with your lack of other symptoms, that would be pretty unlikely. Especially at your age.

DANIELLE: OK, so if I do these tests, what would they be like?

ATTENDING: The CT is like an X-ray. It's literally a two-minute test.

DANIELLE: What kind of radiation exposure are we talking about?

ATTENDING: At our institution, something on the order of 450 X-rays. [Danielle stares at him incredulously.] I know that sounds like a lot, but we do these all the times. It's no big deal, and hopefully the CT will be normal. But sometimes, bleeding in your brain can't be seen on CT. So we need to do a lumbar puncture. That's a bit more involved—

DANIELLE: You mean a spinal tap? [Attending nods.] I'm sorry, but there's no way I can do that. Look, I know you want to be sure I don't have some bad diagnoses, right? But you already said my story doesn't fit for these bad things. I'm sitting here talking to you right now, so how bad could it be? I already feel better. I don't need to do these tests.

ATTENDING: If you feel fine, then why did you come to ER? From what everyone tells me, you weren't feeling so great before. That's why I'd strongly advise you to do the CT as a start. Our job in the ER is to make sure we don't miss life-threatening diagnoses, and yes, they are rare, but we do see cases of subarachnoid hemorrhage in people you might not expect. That's why we have the "subarachnoid pathway." We always do a CT, then if it's a negative, we do a spinal tap.

DANIELLE: Is it an option to do the CT but not the spinal tap?

ATTENDING: Well, it's not our usual protocol. But I suppose it's an option. We can't force you do something you don't want to do. But I would highly advise you to do the lumbar puncture, too. If we are concerned about something this bad, we shouldn't stop halfway. What exactly are you worried about for the spinal tap?

DANIELLE: Well, I hate needles, for one. I'm a pretty big wimp when it comes

---

✚ 911 ACTION TIP

Every test comes with risks. Be sure you know what they are.

✚ 911 ACTION TIP

If you are not comfortable with the diagnostic plan, speak up. You should never feel forced to do something you don't want to do.

---

to pain. I just . . . I would do it if it was really necessary, but I just don't think it is, you know? I feel fine.

ATTENDING: All right, how about this. We can continue to give you IV fluids because it sounds like you were a bit dehydrated, and it's helping you. Once that's done, we can talk again about whether you want to have the CT or lumbar puncture. You already know how I stand on the issue.

DANIELLE: That sounds good. Thank you for being so patient with me. I know it sounds silly, but I just don't want a needle stuck in my back today.

ATTENDING: [chuckles] Makes perfect sense when you put it that way. Do you have any other questions for me?

DANIELLE: Yeah, just . . . Is there any long-term damage from a bad hangover like this?

ATTENDING: I don't think so. I'm not going to tell you it's a good idea to drink so much that you wake up the next morning with a hangover, but, next time, if you *are* drinking alcohol, make sure to drink other fluids as well. That will keep you from getting too dehydrated. And I want you to keep an eye on your symptoms over the next twenty-four hours. Assuming this was just a hangover, you should continue to feel better. If things get worse in any way, I want you to come back and we can have a discussion then about what to do next. OK? [Danielle nods.] And good luck with the rest of your school year.

✚ 911 ACTION TIP

Ask as many questions as you can. Ensure that you understand what is likely to happen with your particular diagnosis.

On one level, the outcome of Danielle's story here doesn't appear to be too different from the original version. In both scenarios, she ended up feeling better and leaving the ER without a lumbar puncture.

But note the significant difference in *how* she left the ER. In the original version, Danielle was so frightened that she pretended to use the bathroom then literally ran from the ER. She probably lost faith in the healthcare system, and if anything had happened and her symptoms worsened, she might not have been willing to return. In the revisited version, she was able to express her concerns, engage in a discussion with the doctor, and reach a working diagnosis and a plan in partnership with her doctor.

What was done differently this time around? First and foremost, Danielle did an excellent job with telling her story, explaining the chronology of events and highlighting her symptoms and which ones worried her (#1). Storytelling is always important, but it is particularly critical when it becomes apparent that other members of the healthcare team may have misunderstood particular elements of a fragmented history. Danielle also expertly redirected the doctor at the point that he was about to walk away in order for her to get "some tests" done (#2).

Take note, also, of how she asked what else he was thinking throughout her history and physical exam and why tests were indicated (#3, 4, 5, 6). By asking these questions, she not only gained knowledge of potential diagnoses, she also established herself as an equal partner in the interaction. Then, she was able to ask about whether she had to follow this "subarachnoid pathway"—instead of blindly following the cookbook approach, she helped come up with a pathway that worked best for her. She was able to have a discussion about the necessity and the risks of the CT scan, and in so doing, avoided the unnecessary radiation, not to mention an invasive and unnecessary spinal tap (#6).

Finally, she kept on coming back to her own common sense diagnosis of this being a hangover (#7), and the doctor eventually agreed with her, working with her to come up with a plan that worked for her (#8). The doctor wouldn't have had to sign her out against medical advice, and she wouldn't have been made to feel trapped and helpless.

May, the Woman Who Fainted at the Sight of a Sandwich

"I don't know about everyone else, but I'm superexcited about this assignment," May told us when we explained this portion of our book to her. "How often do I wish, boy, if I could only do that over, have another shot at it!"

Remember May Gillespie? She was our spunky older lady who passed out at the gym after a workout and a trip to the sauna. ("Let's not forget the smelly fish sandwich," May reminds us.) The doctors were frustrated because she seemed to answer yes to every question. Then she said the magic words, "chest pain," so she got admitted to a cardiology floor. There, she developed a fever, but despite multiple tests, it wasn't until she got very sick, two days into her stay and many tests later, that they figured out what was wrong. By the time they took her to the operating room, her gallbladder was filled with pus and she required a major operation.

Doing over May's story requires a leap of faith: it requires May herself to undergo a significant transformation. One of her defining characteristics is her talkativeness. While her friends and colleagues find her to be hilarious entertainment, this personality feature was also what led the doctors in the original version to label her a "difficult historian" with a "positive review of symptoms." Certainly, the doctors have a duty to get beyond these labels and become better at elucidating the patient's symptoms. At the same time, the patient can also do her part in tailoring the story in a way that highlights key points: timeline, narrative, and context. The worksheets and Prescriptions for Patients illustrate an approach to making sure that important elements of the history are communicated.

Below is an attempt at a "redo." It's a script that we helped to write for May, as a way to show her—and you—how to tell your story and ensure that you are an integral part of the decision-making process.

DOCTOR: Hello, Ms. Gillespie. The paramedics told me about how you fainted at the gym. Did you pass out?

MAY: Hello, doctor. Yes, I did pass out; that's what they tell me at least. Basically, I've been feeling a bit under the weather. I wasn't going to go to the gym, but I thought I should try. I've been going every other day and it's been a pretty good streak. So I was wandering around the gym, feeling

---

+ 911 ACTION TIP

When telling a story, start at the beginning and proceed chronologically, highlighting the parts that are most concerning to you.

---

like "crap," if you'll pardon the expression, and I must have looked like "crap," too, because my two friends came over and said I should sit down. They took me to the sauna. That's where I felt really light-headed. I tried to stand up to get out of the hot air, but then I saw these bright spots dancing in front of my eyes. I think that's when I fell to the ground. Everyone sounded so far away. . . . My friends tried to help me up, then one of them gave me this really awful-smelling sandwich. That's when I passed out again. Next thing I knew I was in an ambulance, and now here I am.

DOCTOR: So when exactly would you say your symptoms started?

MAY: The fainting and things, that was all today. But I haven't been feeling right for a week or so. Everyone's been coming down with something, so I didn't think much of it.

DOCTOR: Have you been sneezing and coughing?

MAY: No, not really. It's more that I've had some stomach issues. Nothing big, just some cramping pains once in a while. I've also had body aches and no appetite at all.

DOCTOR: Any fever? Recent travel?

MAY: Maybe I felt warm, but I didn't measure it. No travel, nothing south of Connecticut.

DOCTOR: Can you tell me if you have pain in any particular part of your belly?

MAY: No, I think it's kind of all over. But I can show you better where it hurts most to push.

DOCTOR: Sure. But before we go there, tell me more about the chest pains. The paramedics said that you were having some chest pains at the gym?

MAY: [pausing] Well, I'm not sure it was really chest pain. It was kind of high on my belly. And it really wasn't that bad unless I tried to eat anything.

DOCTOR: OK, so you were having belly pain. Then you passed out?

+ 911 ACTION TIP

Clarify your symptoms with your doctor. Put them in context.

MAY: Actually, we went into the sauna. Me and my friends. After about five minutes, I was feeling worse. I tried to stand up and I got all woozy.

DOCTOR: At any point, were you having chest palpitations? Or any trouble breathing?

MAY: No, nothing like that. [pauses] Why do you ask?

DOCTOR: I'm trying to figure out what caused your syncope. We need to make sure it wasn't a cardiac etiology.

MAY: I'm sorry, doctor, but I'm not certain I understand what you're saying. Do you mind explaining to me what you mean by "syncope" and "cardiac etiology"?

DOCTOR: Sorry. Let me try again. In someone your age who passed out, we always think about a heart rhythm issue, or a heart attack, and we need to make sure it's not any of those scary things.

MAY: I've never been told I have heart problems. Is this what a heart attack feels like?

DOCTOR: [looking at EKG in the chart] Well, the good news is that the heart tracing that the medics did on your way over here looks pretty good. I don't see any abnormal rhythm or obvious signs of heart damage.

MAY: Well, that is good news! Is there anything else you're worried about?

DOCTOR: Sure. We also think about neurological causes, and make sure it's not a stroke, for example. Other things we have to "rule out" in our minds include aortic dissection and pulmonary embolism.

MAY: Sounds scary. What about my stomach not feeling right—could that be related to anything?

DOCTOR: Well, it's hard to say—

+ 911 ACTION TIP

Ask your doctor to explain if he uses words that you don't understand.

✚ 911 ACTION TIP

Engage your doctor in the differential diagnosis as you go through your narrative. Offer up connections that you see as relevant.

✚ 911 ACTION TIP

Let your doctor know that it's OK if she doesn't know exactly what you have. You still want to hear her impressions and her thought process.

MAY: I'm not saying you have to be 100 percent sure. I just want to know what you think might be going on, given what you've heard so far.

DOCTOR: Well, if I have to guess . . . I'd say you might have two different processes going on, too. Say you had a stomach bug. That made you feel weaker and dehydrated. Then you fainted because you were dehydrated and hot, and had what we call a vaso-vagal episode. That's what I suspect happened.

MAY: Is there anything else you can think of? I've had stomach bugs before but I've never fainted with them.

DOCTOR: Sure, there's a ton of possibilities. We may be able to narrow things down a bit after I've examined you.

MAY: OK. Would you mind pointing out what you're looking for as we go along?

DOCTOR: Of course. [He listens to her heart and lungs.] Your heart and lungs sound pretty normal. No sign of pneumonia. I do hear a click in your heart. Have you been told that you have mitral valve prolapse before?

MAY: Oh yes, many years ago. They said it's nothing to worry about.

DOCTOR: Absolutely. I'm just pointing it out, as you asked. [He begins to feel her belly.] Does this hurt anywhere?

MAY: [wincing] Right there. It does hurt.

DOCTOR: Hmm. That area is right over your gallbladder. Have you had any surgeries in your belly before?

MAY: I had a hysterectomy years ago. Nothing else.

DOCTOR: Any trouble with your gallbladder before?

MAY: No, not that I know of. I've had a lot of what I call "indigestion" over the past few months, though.

DOCTOR: Yes. Well, we'll do some tests looking at your gallbladder, too—an ultrasound and a CT scan—plus we'll see what your labs show. But also we shouldn't forget the other things we talked about, just to be sure. I definitely want to keep you on the heart monitor for now.

MAY: That sure is a lot of tests. . . . I've heard that getting a CT scan is like living through Hiroshima, it's that much radiation. Do you really think the CT would add a lot more to all those other tests?

DOCTOR: It does provide some additional information, yes, especially if we're concerned about your appendix or any other infection of your intestines.

MAY: But you didn't say those were the things you were most worried about.

DOCTOR: OK, how about this? Let's do the blood work and ultrasound first. If the ultrasound turns up something, we can stop there. If the ultrasound doesn't show anything, we can move on to the CT scan.

MAY: That sounds good. Oh, before I forget to mention, I thought about my gallbladder because for the past week, it's hurt the worst whenever I tried to eat. I remember before my sister had hers out, they told her to avoid greasy foods. Do you think that still fits in with what we're discussing?

DOCTOR: Actually, yes, that does make sense. I still think the heart warrants close attention, and we can't be sure if it's not something else all together, but the gallbladder ties everything together the best.

✚ 911 ACTION TIP

What tests you get should make sense to you. If it doesn't, ask.

✚ 911 ACTION TIP

Perform a final common sense check of the working diagnosis.

MAY: Thanks for explaining, doctor. And in the meantime, is there anything we can do to make me feel better?

DOCTOR: Of course. Let's start with some fluids and some medicine for nausea, and see how you're feeling when the tests come back.

We showed these revised scenarios to a group of our patients. Some were impressed. Others told us that these read like fairy tales.

"No way I could sound that cool and collected," one of them said. "I can't tell a story like that on a good day, much less if I'd just passed out and found myself lying in a stretcher in an ER!"

It's true that in situations where you are highly stressed, it is hard to pull yourself together and think about strategies for telling a good story or inserting yourself into conversations at the right places. This is why it's so important to do the work now. You need to practice and be ready. Before your faculties are stretched to the limit in a difficult and painful situation, take the time, at home, at work, with your family and friends, to develop the skills you need. That way, when it matters the most, you will be an expert at advocating for your own health.

In the redone scenario, the coherent, step-wise story that May "told" allowed the doctor to pick up abdominal pain as being critical to the diagnosis. This is in stark contrast to the original rambling version that led the attending to virtually abandon May to a medical student, then pigeonholing her with a label of "syncope" and "chest pain." The doctor's approach in the original scenario was hardly admirable, but there are specific things to do to avoid eliciting such a reaction. Straightforward storytelling—Pillar #1—is the way to go.

In the revised version, May also advocated for her being part of the thought process (#2), challenging the assumptions about a "cardiac" problem and advancing her own theory about what happened. Notice how she made sure she was involved in the critical portions of the physical exam (#3), and the ease at which the doctor discussed the issue of the heart murmur with her. Her being so open to a two-way dialogue also helped the doctor develop a comfort with her to ask about pain with the abdominal exam, which turned out to be a critical clue to her overall diagnosis.

Going on to Pillar #4, May was persistent in thinking through her differential diagnosis. In this case, the doctor responded positively. Still, she asked if there was anything else that could have been forgotten, in a non-confrontational way that elicited a positive reaction from the doctor. Note how the initial diagnostic momentum focusing on cardiac causes changed as a result of questions she asked to broaden the differential diagnosis.

At the end of the physical exam, May had established herself as an equal partner in the diagnostic process (#5). She asked about the necessity and risks of testing, and together, she and her doctor decided about next steps and which tests to get and when (#6). Then, she had one last common sense check when she asked about some other symptoms that she had forgotten to mention earlier (#7). Was there any chance the new symptoms could bring about a diagnosis they hadn't thought of yet? In fact, the symptoms fit into the working diagnosis well, which led further away from "ruling out" heart problems that had plagued the original version. It's obvious, then, how May and her doctor were able to integrate diagnosis into the healing process (#8). In this redone version, May could have been diagnosed with a gallbladder infection straight away. She would have started to feel better physically and emotionally, and would have avoided the agony, uncertainty, and complications associated with the delay in diagnosis.

Every patient in our focus group agreed that they can learn from the revised scripts, and without question, everyone liked the new version better than the original one. Some, though, argued that the comparison isn't fair. "In the original version, Jerry, Annette, Danielle, and May all got doctors who practiced cookbook medicine," they complained. "Compare that to the new version, where they got better doctors who knew about partnership and really worked to involve their patients in diagnosis."

Or did they? In the revisited versions, the doctors started out with the same predictable, cookbook patterns as before. It was Jerry, Annette, Danielle, and May who changed their approach. Read this chapter again if you don't believe us. Count the number of dichotomous, close-ended questions these doctors asked, and the number of times they interrupted their patients' narratives. Look how early the doctor fixated on what they thought was the "chief complaint." Recognize how attention was focused on "ruling out" and "working up" the "worst-case scenario." See how quickly the doctor brought out the "pathway." Count the number of times they tried to end the conversation before the patient was ready. These doctors are the same cookbook doctors as before. It was only with careful guidance from their patients that the doctors began to respond accordingly, in a more thoughtful, reflective, and collaborative way.

We would love to have doctors initiate the 8 Pillars and practice this patient-centered approach on their own accord. This will not happen overnight, and chances are, the next time you see a doctor, you will detect the cookbook style that you recognize well by now. The power to change lies with you: you can't reform the entire medical establishment by yourself overnight, but you can arm yourself with the tools you need to get the care you deserve. You can encourage your doctor along the process of getting the right diagnosis for you, and make all the difference to your medical care.

911 REVIEW

- Patient outcomes can be dramatically different when the 8 Pillars to Better Diagnosis are practiced.
- Your doctor may be schooled in cookbook medicine, but you have the ability to change your medical care.
- Practice the 8 Pillars today. You will see a dramatic impact on your next interaction with your doctor.

Part V

Prescription for Reform

In the final two chapters, we demonstrate the potential impact of our approach on the larger scale. Chapter 16 shows how aiming for the right diagnosis for the individual patient can have long-ranging effects on the overall healthcare system. Chapter 17 illustrates how diagnostic partnership can work in the real world, and demonstrates how it can be applied, every day, by patients and by doctors, by believers and by skeptics.

Sixteen

Diagnosis, Multiplied

A businessman, a public defender, and a grocer are running for office. They are each asked a question: "What's the biggest problem facing healthcare in the United States?"

"That's easy," says the businessman. "It's too expensive. We spend more per capita on healthcare than any other country."

"There's a bigger problem than that!" exclaims the public defender. "There are 50 million people in the United States who don't have health insurance. We need to make sure everyone has access to healthcare."

"How are you going to pay for these extra people without spending even more?" the businessman counters. "Our healthcare system is broken and can't be stretched anymore. We already have a huge deficit going; that's Chinese dollars we're spending."

The grocer clears his throat. "Actually, I think the biggest problem with the U.S. healthcare system is obesity."

There is a long silence. The grocer continues. "I'm not talking about obese *people*—that's another story. I'm talking about an obese *system*. Patients, doctors, hospitals: everybody thinks more is better. Take my customers. I see them getting fatter and fatter. And why is that? It's because we offer them an overabundance of food at low up-front cost. Customers are happy. I make money. People buy more, eat more, and worry later. It's the same with our healthcare system. Unless something changes, the system just keeps growing and growing, getting fatter and fatter. That's the obesity epidemic exemplified in our healthcare system."

The grocer wins our vote. There are signs of profligate use of healthcare resources everywhere we look. CTs are ordered for small head bumps; stress tests are ordered as routine exams; tests of questionable benefit are promulgated as the latest and greatest—only to be retracted when evidence comes out to the contrary and these tests are quickly replaced by the next, latest and greatest advance.[1] Unnecessary testing alone is estimated to cost up to $250 billion extra each year.[2] Our healthcare system has become morbidly obese: there are too many tests done too often without justification, and our system has become too expensive and too inefficient.

Those without access to care obviously suffer the most. But those who have access to every resource aren't getting the best care, either. There is a belief that getting the best care means getting the most care, but very often, more is just more, not better.

What America needs is the *right* medical care, care that is leaner and more patient-centered, starting with the right diagnosis and leading to the right treatment. In this chapter, we demonstrate how the concepts of the partnership approach and the emphasis on diagnosis form the basis for meaningful healthcare reform. We show how the grocer hit the nail on the head: healthcare in the United States isn't the best, but it sure is the fattest. We illustrate how improving care for you and partnering toward your own diagnosis is the first, most essential step toward fixing our broken healthcare system.

In the wake of the economic recession, thousands of young people had trouble finding jobs. Twenty-four-year-old Tim Johnson was one of them. Five years earlier, he had chosen Babson College, a school well known for its business programs, over his local public university because it seemed like the world of opportunity would be open to him.

"When I was looking at schools, all the Babson grads were finding jobs in top consulting firms and investment banks," he tells us.

Unfortunately, it was a different story by the time he graduated. Even though he maintained a 3.5 GPA and had two summer internships under his belt, he had trouble finding a job. More than a year after he finished college, he was bartending at a local pub while trying to make some extra money as a math tutor.

"It's OK," he shruggs. "I mean, I was hoping to find a job in marketing, but at least I can make ends meet."

He saved money by living with his boyfriend. His parents helped him out with his college loan payments. Because he was healthy, one thing he didn't worry about was health insurance. He hadn't needed it—until one day, when he started having severe abdominal cramping.

"It started so suddenly. I had just woken up and was eating some cereal. Then I almost doubled over because of the pain. It felt like a terrible cramp on the right side of my abdomen—like gas, but much worse. I got up and tried moving around, but it wouldn't go away. I even tried going to the bathroom. It was so bad, I thought I was going to pass out." It took half an hour to get in touch with his partner, Aaron, who promptly came home and brought him to the ER.

The pain was a little better by the time he got to the ER but it was still severe. "To the ER's credit, they took my symptoms seriously. A doctor came to see me right away when I got there. He asked me a few questions, pressed on my belly, and then asked a nurse to put in an IV and give me some medications for pain."

Tim was told that they would need to get "abdominal labs" and a CT scan.

"What do you think it is?" he asked nervously.

"I'm not sure," the doctor said. "It could be a lot of things. Appendicitis, kidney stones—we have to consider all these things. We'll start with some blood tests, but we'll need a CT scan to find out for sure. If you use the bathroom, let the nurse know so we can get a urine and stool sample, too."

Tim and Aaron looked at each other. "Wow, that sounds like a lot of tests," Tim said. "Any idea how much it would cost? I don't have insurance—"

"You shouldn't think about cost," Aaron cut in. "If you need to do it, we'll make it work."

The doctor was nodding. "Your friend is right: you can't be thinking about money when it could cost you your life."

So Tim had his blood drawn. He produced some urine and handed the specimen cup to one of the techs. He waited for his CT scan, and then for the result. His pain got worse again, but after some pain medications, he felt better.

"Good news!" The doctor appeared, smiling. "We didn't find anything on the CT scan! Your appendix looks fine. You don't have any kidney stones. You can go ahead and get dressed; we'll have your discharge paperwork ready in just a few minutes."

Tim frowned. "So what is it? What do I have?"

"I'm not sure," came the reply. "I don't think it's anything serious. Maybe you're just constipated. The CT scan did show a lot of stool in your colon."

Tim was not convinced. "I knew what it felt like to be constipated; I've been constipated before," he tells us later. "This wasn't constipation! No one bothered to ask me, but I've been having regular bowel movements all week—that morning included. You'd think after all the tests they ran, they could have come up with something better than 'constipation.' I was beyond frustrated, but I felt hopeless to do anything about it."

Tim's exasperation was obvious to everyone in the ER; that, and the fact that his pain was starting to come back worse than ever, persuaded the ER doctor to ask for a surgical consult. Before long, a team of surgeons came into his room and pressed on his belly some more. This time, they also had him pull down his boxer shorts for what seemed like a hernia exam, except that he wasn't asked to cough. There was some discussion about his right testicle and then a stern, older gentleman who introduced himself as the attending surgeon mentioned the possibility of needing an operation.

Tim didn't understand. An hour earlier, the ER doctor was talking about sending him going home. Now he has to have an operation on his testicle? "I want a second opinion!"

Dr. Kosowsky: I happened to be on call that day, and was told about an angry patient who was about to sign out against medical advice. When I arrived, I could tell that Tim and his partner were upset and confused. I would have been, too, if I had been in their position. So I decided to start from the beginning, with the story that brought Tim to the ER in the first place. Almost immediately, it became clear: abrupt onset of severe pain in the lower abdomen; nothing remarkable on abdominal exam; a normal abdominal

CT scan. The clue was not to be found in the abdomen, because Tim had testicular torsion: a very dangerous condition that occurs when the testicle twists on itself, cutting off blood supply and causing excruciating pain as the testicle tissue dies.

Dr. Wen: I don't understand . . . why didn't he have a testicular exam in the first place?

Dr. Kosowsky: Patients with torsion tend to have pain in the testicles, but it's sometimes overshadowed by "referred pain" to the abdomen—pain is felt in the abdomen instead of the testicles. This has to do with the way the male genito-urinary system develops and how the nerve fibers to the testicle remain connected after birth. In any case, there aren't too many things that can cause sudden, severe pain on one side of the abdomen, and testicular torsion is one of them. In this case, the doctors were relying on the wrong diagnostic tests. Torsion can't be found by blood tests and CT scans of the abdomen; it's clinical diagnosis, based on history and physical exam.[3]

Dr. Wen: And that's why forming a differential diagnosis is so important! So what happened to Tim?

Dr. Kosowsky: I had a conversation with Tim and his partner, and I answered a lot of their questions. From that point on, the treatment course was clear. Tim went to the operating room, but unfortunately, his testicle had to be removed because there had been no blood flow for some time and it was no longer viable.

Dr. Wen: That's another remarkable example of how a shotgun approach to testing comes at a real cost. I'm not talking about the dollar cost here (though no doubt doing the shotgun approach is certainly expensive): blindly going through tests won't get you to the right diagnosis, and that can have terrible consequences for patients.

We didn't come up with our approach to diagnosis in order to save on costs—we advocate for it because it can lead to better care. Cost savings are a by-product, something that just happens to follow when medicine is practiced in a more thoughtful way. Think about the extra costs accrued for Jerry with his hospital stay and stress test, or Arthur with his multiple brain scans: we are talking tens of thousands of dollars. Our healthcare system is opaque, so most of these costs aren't paid directly by patients, but someone is paying for the extra care—extra care that does not translate to better care.

Doctors and politicians alike have become afraid to talk about cost. There are many people who will point to any discussion about cutting cost as "rationing," which is a dirty word in this country. Every expenditure has to come out of someone's lunch bucket, and any time there is a discussion of cost-cutting, there will be some accusation of doing less for patients just to save money. This runs counter to the American mentality that we want to get the most healthcare possible for ourselves, especially when we're not paying for it directly.

What these people don't realize is that, a lot of the time, extra care is actually worse care. Think about Denise Valiant and Fiona McCloskey and the negative consequences of getting unnecessary tests and procedures. They both had hospital bills amounting to the tens of thousands of dollars, with a negative impact on their health. Or take May Gillespie and the many tests she had in the hospital without getting to the right diagnosis. The issue here wasn't the number of tests per se or the cost of these tests: it was that there was a significant delay to getting the *right* test and the *right* diagnosis. The same thing for Tim Johnson, whose providers failed to do the *right* test on him and totally missed the boat on his diagnosis.

Our medical system is broken because it doesn't incentivize doctors to arrive at the correct diagnosis. In fact, perverse economic incentives exist such that doctors are often reimbursed *more* for ordering more tests. There are also entire industries that depend on more tests, more procedures, and more (potentially wrong) treatments to make profit. It's to their advantage to "rule out" unlikely diagnoses with extra tests and "workups" when a simple history and personal exam would often suffice. (Though these companies are unlikely to oppose our common sense approach to patient care; who would admit that they do not support using a tailored, individualized approach that aims to get to the right diagnosis?)

At the moment, entities that should support cost-cutting are promoting strategies that do not work. Third-party payers like Medicare Medicaid and private insurers, have strong incentives to keep costs down, but their mandated rules, restrictions, and approval processes end up being counter-productive. Ironically, these entities that have the strongest economic incentives to cut costs are some of the major influences to promote cookbook medicine, which actually is the root cause of excessive testing and skyrocketing costs.

As a society, we have to get away from incentives that promote unnecessary care, but the way to do it isn't to impose recipes on individual patients. The solution to better care is thoughtful, individualized care that begins with the patient and his or her doctor. Patients need to make sure their stories are being heard and engage with their doctors in the differential diagnosis *before* any tests are ordered. They should resist submitting to random, shotgun tests. They should always leave with a working diagnosis. This is particularly important if the patient is going home and this is their one opportunity to see a doctor, but it's also important for the patient who is being admitted to the hospital—why delay your diagnosis and feel bad for longer?

Ultimately, we need to trim down the obesity in our system—but not through irrational and capricious cost-cutting. With the approach that we advocate, we emphasize that diagnosis is the lynchpin to better healthcare. Reform efforts need to have the goal of developing a leaner, more efficient system, and this all starts with getting patients the right diagnosis. With the move away from fee-for-service payments and the emergence of new concepts like the Accountable Care Organizations, we may be starting to see some of the perverse incentives overturned. This may be a good way forward for the nation overall, but at the end of the day, we believe that everything has to start with the individual patient. Doctors and patients both have to work toward an individualized, diagnosis-oriented, and common sense approach to medical care. This is what will transform our healthcare system.

So what does this ideal medical care look like?

The great Tip O'Neill, himself a Boston man, used to say, "All politics is local." We believe in its corollary, that all medicine is personal. The world of better medicine starts with the individual patient interacting with the individual doctor.

In this world, the patient receives tailored care in partnership with her doctor. She gets a version of "personalized medicine" where her unique narrative forms the basis of her history and subsequent physical exam. Doctor and patient work together to build a personalized differential diagnosis and develop a personalized plan to move forward. Together, they reach a working diagnosis. The patient's value systems are explored and taken into consideration in considering treatment options.

In this world, the patient receives a more efficient, more accurate diagnosis. There are fewer tests ordered, because instead of a shotgun or cookbook approach, tests are done with specific indications in mind. Fewer tests mean fewer abnormal results, fewer procedures, and fewer avoidable complications.

As a result of knowing her diagnosis, the patient will have a better understanding of how to approach her disease. She will feel more committed to moving forward with the treatments. She will understand the natural history of her condition, and learn what steps can be taken to alter the course and alleviate the symptoms. She will feel better as a result of having seen her doctor.

A closer partnership will save time, both for the patient and the doctor. As for malpractice, we already know that better communication decreases the chance of malpractice litigation. Our hope is that this way of practicing medicine will reduce malpractice suits, because patients and doctors will work closely together and always in the patient's best interest. Doctors will stop perceiving patients as dangerous adversaries, and patients will stop being afraid to ask their doctors questions.

In this world, the patient will continue on the path to becoming more savvy about healthcare decisions. She will share in the doctor's thought process and always think about the differential diagnosis. She will help her doctor narrow down the differential diagnosis to one or two working diagnoses, and begin the healing from there. This will extend from diagnosis into the treatment realms, which already have excellent movements toward shared decision-making in considering the ultimate course of treatments. As this transformation in medicine takes place, and as evidence accumulates showing that more aggressive and more costly care doesn't equate to better care,[5] the patient will adjust her expectations and learn to ask for better—not more—treatments.

The notion of patient-centered and individualized medicine extends far beyond the diagnostic partnership to many other issues in the healthcare reform debate. For example, much has been written about the cost of end-of-life care: does it make sense that 40 percent of a person's total lifetime expenditure in health comes during the last year of their life—up to $145,000 per person? Dr. Daniel Callahan and Dr. Sherwin Nuland wrote an excellent editorial on our society's struggle with accepting death and dying, and how it is time for us to spend more energy trying to improve the quality of life rather than do everything possible to fight off death.[4] These are all questions our society should task ourselves with answering.

Doctoring is about care of the individual patient. Healthcare reform is about systems—but in order for the system to be fixed, it must start with the individual patient and the individual doctor.

Our goal is not to ration healthcare, and this book is not a primer on how to cut costs. What it does aim to do is to improve healthcare for each person, each reader, each patient. What it does strive for is to demonstrate the integral role that diagnosis plays in leading to better care. Our book is about you, about helping you establish a partnership with your doctor and work toward diagnosis on your way to better treatment and a better life.

We also believe that what is good for the individual is good for the country. Stop unnecessary tests in favor of focusing on the diagnosis. Cut the cookbook recipes, the "rule-out" and the "pathways" in favor of a thoughtful, common sense, and individualized approach to medicine. End the obesity in our healthcare system in favor of better, leaner medical care. This is our prescription for better healthcare for you and for the United States healthcare system.

911 REVIEW

- The U.S. is suffering from an obesity epidemic when it comes to healthcare. Excessive care is often just that, and it leads to worse outcomes, unnecessary testing, and unhappy patients.
- Many efforts aimed at cutting costs have resulted only in more cookbook recipes, which do, paradoxically, form the root of our dysfunctional health system.
- Better care begins with focusing on the individual patient. Instead of more recipes to cut costs, focus on tailored, patient-centered care and aim for the diagnosis.
- Reforming your healthcare is the first and most critical step to healthcare reform for the nation.

Seventeen

Countering the Skeptics

We are idealists who strongly advocate for the principles of an individualized, patient-centered approach to healthcare. We are realists, too; we recognize that there will be opposition to any attempt to overhaul the status quo that is cookbook medicine. Campaigning for reform generates controversy; proposing change elicits defensiveness.

In this chapter, we address the critics and counter the skeptics by answering eight "frequently asked questions." We draw upon our own experiences and those of expert medical voices to provide answers to these questions. Our critics will question how our vision for the patient-physician partnership can work in the real world; this chapter shows them how.

"In railing against overtesting, aren't you advocating for a return to the Dark Ages? Shouldn't we be taking advantage of science and technology, not running away from it?"

We agree that scientific progress holds tremendous potential for advancing the quality of healthcare. In the preceding chapters, we have cited numerous examples of how these new technologies have enhanced our ability to make diagnoses and improve the lives of our patients. We're not Luddites; in no way are we advocating a return to entrails and divining rods.

However, subservience to technology is not the answer, either. Dr. Howard Blumstein, a practicing emergency physician in North Carolina, is the immediate past president of the American Academy of Emergency Medicine. He refers to our overreliance on diagnostic technologies as "diagnostic creep":

"It used to be that before ordering a simple X-ray, we would really think about what we need the test for and how the results will change the patient's management," he says. "Now, it's become so easy to order a CT that I hear doctors say, 'I'm just going to order the CT because I want to be sure I don't miss anything.' Ordering tests has become a knee-jerk reaction; doctors stop thinking about what they're being used for, and then these tests take a life of their own. Often, it's not in the patient's best interest, because there's false reassurance when nothing shows up and confusion and anxiety around incidental findings that require follow-up. Not to mention the radiation risk, which I think is just inexcusable unless you really have a good reason for ordering that CT scan."

The bottom line is that, when used right, technology can save lives. But cookbook thinking and practice results in a misplaced dependence on technology, with decisions being made by reflex rather than through reflection. This is the aspect of technology that we take issue with and seek to reform. Ultimately, our opposition is not to technology, but to technology supplanting rational, common sense decision-making.

"In the real world, patients expect to have tests done. Think about the commercials for the total body 'health scans,' and the 'diagnostic centers' popping up in malls around the country. In our society, patients are conditioned to believe that more is better."

One of the many good things about the consumer movement in healthcare is that more patients are taking an active role in advocating for what they believe to be in their best interest.[1] When patients are asking for specific tests, they are simply demonstrating a desire to be engaged in the diagnostic process, as they understand it. In our experience, most patients aren't asking for testing for the sake of testing; they just want to find out what, if anything, is wrong with them. Unfortunately, their trust in technology is often greater than their trust in doctors. But we believe that a critical ele-

ment of doctoring is a commitment to the diagnostic process as a partnership; and part of that partnership involves teaching patients about the
appropriate role of testing.

For the patient who does come in requesting a specific test, the doctor
first needs to find out what's driving the request: is it based on personal
experience? ("Whenever I have a cough they always order a chest X-ray.")
Something they saw on TV? ("I saw an ad for a total body scan.") Someone
else's experience? ("A friend of mine was having headaches, and her MRI
showed a brain tumor.") The advice of another health-care professional? ("I
spoke to my doctor over the phone, and he told me to go to the ER for a CT
scan.") Sometimes the request makes sense; if so, the doctor should be able to
understand why. If not, then the first and most important step is a discussion
with the patient. Initially, patients may seem mollified by reflex testing, but
our experience suggests that when patients work together with their doctor
through the process of differential diagnosis (rather than through arbitrary
and potentially harmful tests), they are far more satisfied.[2]

Dr. Ali Raja agrees with us. A physician at Brigham and Women's Hospital and an assistant professor at Harvard Medical School, Dr. Raja points
out that for every study that suggests that patients want more testing, there
are studies showing that patient satisfaction is actually highest when the patient is involved in the diagnosis. And, importantly, a more engaged patient
is more likely to follow through with their treatment regimen and experience a better outcome.

"That makes sense, right?" he asks. "Say I'm taking care of a patient who
fell and hit his head, has a headache, and wants a CT scan. I can see the patient for thirty seconds and order a CT scan of his head. If it's negative, then
I'll send him home. I gave the patient what he thought he wanted, so you
think he would be happy. However, at the end of his visit, my patient would
still have no idea what the scan was done to evaluate for why he continues
to have a headache, and what to do about it."

So Dr. Raja has a different approach. "What if I take ten minutes to talk
to him? I can ask about his symptoms and do a careful exam. We can discuss the differential diagnosis for headaches and explore whether a head
CT will be useful in making a diagnosis. I can explain to him that I think
he most likely has a concussion, and why I don't think a head CT is useful

in making that diagnosis. I can talk about what he should expect over the coming days and how to improve these symptoms. The patient will feel more satisfied and more empowered after this conversation because he will understand my thought process, and will have participated in the decision-making process. He may still have a headache, but this is not going to be a patient who is going to go home and be confused and unhappy about his care."

Dr. Ron Walls, professor and chair of emergency medicine at the Brigham and Women's Hospitals, refers to medical testing as "the intrusion of potentially expensive and lengthy processes into the care of the patient." Therefore, he says, it is imperative that doctors know the question before they order the test, rather than ordering it as a reflex or as a substitute for spending the time exploring the precise details of the patient's history at the bedside.

"There is often an intellectual laziness on the part of doctors, who misguidedly rely on testing and 'numbers' when what is really needed is to take a good history," says Dr. Walls. "Doctors are eager to jump to testing. But testing is a double-edged sword. A lot of times, tests will add nothing at all and might even provide false assurance, or a misleading direction."

Dr. Walls and Dr. Raja agree with us that doctors need to do a better job of explaining the pros and cons of testing, and in particular, explaining the risks associated with tests. Tests cost money, they take time, and they can have side effects like radiation exposure.[3] Ultimately, it's not about saving time or money, but about working in the patient's best interest. Patients whose doctors are committed to partnering with them through the diagnostic process are unlikely to demand something that sounded appealing based on a commercial.[4]

"The kind of medicine you advocate for takes time to practice. Doctors today are busier than they've ever been, and patients, too, are impatient and want their answer right away. Is your approach compatible with the fast pace of modern medicine?"

Practicing an individualized, patient-centered approach to medicine does take an upfront investment of time. It requires the doctor to sit down with the patient and carefully go through the history and physical, and then have a discussion about differential diagnosis, and likelihoods, and pros and cons of testing. But does it actually take up more time overall?

Nobody has done a study about this, so this is our hypothesis: we believe that our approach to medical care actually saves time in aggregate, for both the patient and the doctor. With cookbook practice, the patient may have to wait for hours to get laboratory tests back and CT scans done, the results of which are, more often than not, unrevealing and probably wouldn't have made their diagnosis or changed their management. A discussion up front saves the time that would have been wasted with test after test in pursuit of one "rule-out" after another—and perhaps, another diagnosis could have been discovered that would have otherwise taken months to uncover.

From the doctor's standpoint, it may seem like taking the time to engage with each patient is incompatible with modern-day practice. In the final analysis, though, arriving at a working diagnosis on the first go-around is what saves time. In addition, instead of having to follow up on tests and wondering what to do with abnormal results, the doctor who uses tests thoughtfully and sparingly can spend time partnering with her patient around decisions that really matter. In this way, quality and efficiency go hand in hand.[5]

Expert doctors will tell you that listening carefully to the patient narrative saves time for them in the end. "Doctors roll their eyes and think, gosh, if I let my patient go on and on, I'll just spend my whole day listening to Aunt Tilly," says Dr. Lisa Sanders, an internist at Yale and the medical adviser to *House, M.D.* "But I've found that when I let my patients talk, their story takes just as long as if I bombard them with random questions."

Dr. Walls concurs. "It may seem easier for the doctor to rush through the history and then compensate by ordering tests, but this doesn't save time. In reality, it is a false economy, because the tests add hours to the patient's visit, while other patients are backed up in the waiting room, thus delaying care and prolonging their visits also. While appropriate testing is essential to accurate diagnosis, unnecessary tests just add cost and inefficiency, which we can avoid by really listening to our patients and spending the time with them up front."

As to whether it is feasible to practice this patient-centered approach in a variety of medical settings, we refer back to what we said in our introduction: if we can incorporate it in the fast-paced, high-patient volume setting of the ER, then the primary care doctor can do it in his office practice, too. So can the specialist in the clinic, the hospitalist on the ward, or the intensive care doctor in the ICU. If we can aim for diagnosis in the ER setting, having never met the patient before, with limited time and under high-stress environments, then truly any doctor can, too.

"You always talk about the importance of diagnosis. But you said yourselves: it's rare that a doctor can be 100 percent confident of it. So is the doctor supposed to pretend? Why not just say that the patient has an unexplained symptom, like 'headache' or 'chest pain,' rather than speculating about the unknown?"

We believe that diagnosis is the key to good healthcare: without a diagnosis, patients (and their doctors) can't know what to expect, and treatment priorities have no context. This doesn't mean that the process of arriving at a diagnosis is always straightforward. Actually, we think that the pursuit of diagnosis is one of the most challenging and fulfilling aspects of medicine.

So what to do if the patient's diagnosis is not 100 percent clear? Here's what we would advise doctors: tell your patient! Let's say that a patient has a headache. We are pretty sure based on the patient's description of it that it's a migraine, but can we be 100 percent certain? No, because there is a chance it could be a tension headache, or pain that comes from the eyes, or a sinus infection; theoretically, the headache could also be from a brain tumor, a stroke, or meningitis. All of these possibilities together form the differential diagnosis for the patient's headache.

If this were our patient, we would explain the differential diagnosis to him. We would run through the possibilities and comment on the likelihood of each: migraine is likely, based on the headache features and prior history; sinus infection is less likely because the following signs and symptoms are not present; there is nothing to suggest a brain tumor or stroke, and here are reasons why. We can't necessarily provide the diagnosis of migraine with 100 percent certainty, but we can work through the differential diagnosis and talk about our options going forward: whether we're close enough to a working diagnosis that further testing won't add much; whether the consequences of missing a particular diagnosis warrant a specific test to narrow down the differential diagnosis; whether we are confident enough in our working diagnosis that we can predict an expected course and/or treatment options.

At the end of the day, we won't send our patient home unless we are reasonably reassured that he will be OK. That's our job as doctors. Equally important, our patient will understand what the natural course of his headache
is expected to be and what treatments should make his symptoms improve.
He will also have a better appreciation of what other diagnoses are out
there, including a diagnosis we may have missed; he will know what things
to look out for and what not to worry about. And if there was a particular
diagnosis he was concerned about (say he had a childhood friend who died
of a brain tumor), his concerns will have been addressed.

Doesn't this process sound infinitely better than a generic "headache
pathway" that comes from a cookbook recipe that rarely actually gets you
to a diagnosis? Isn't this better than being told that your diagnosis is the very
symptom you came to the doctor having? Except in rare circumstances,[6] being given a diagnosis of "I don't know" isn't satisfactory for the patient or the
doctor.

You know by now that we are not fans of the "rule-outs" or "pathways,"
but this also doesn't mean that we want doctors to make up a diagnosis or
force a square peg into a round hole when the diagnosis doesn't really make
sense. (Remember the hazards that come from forcing a diagnosis to fit the
presentation!) Rather, the approach we advocate for is to carefully consider
the differential diagnosis and narrow it down to the most likely disease that
explains the patient's symptoms, while making sure that the patient understands and is engaged in the entire diagnostic process.

*"Cutting down on tests is fraught with medico-legal liability for doctors.
Won't doctors be sued more?"*

We hear this argument all the time, but we don't understand the logic.
Study after study has demonstrated that lawsuits happen when there is poor
communication, not when there is lack of testing. Interviews with patients
and family members who have sued their doctors reveal common themes:
"the doctor didn't take my concerns seriously," "the doctor didn't take the
time to hear what I was trying to tell him," and "the doctor never told me
what was going on with all the tests." It's the detached and impersonal
"workup" that gets doctors into trouble. On the other hand, a patient-
centered approach, where the patient is listened to, the differential diagnosis

is tailored to the patient and decisions are made together, is less likely to result in legal action. Not to mention, careful attention to the patient's story and a collaborative approach to diagnosis will also increase the chances of getting to the right diagnosis and so decrease the likelihood of ending up with a bad outcome.

Ohio physician Dr. Michael Weinstock is the coauthor of the popular Bouncebacks! series of books and podcasts that explores cases where patients are misdiagnosed on their first visit to the ER, and end up returning a day or two later, often in worse condition.[7] He acknowledges that many physicians order tests as a way to try to cover themselves.

"What they're trying to do is to balance the short-term risk of litigation to themselves against the long-term health of the patient," he says. "Right now, our litigation system is not one that punishes the doctor for excessive tests that cause harm. So doctors are not thinking, if I get this CT of their neck now, could they have health effects like thyroid cancer later in their life. They're only thinking, I hope I don't get sued because I missed a freak neck fracture."

But does ordering more tests actually lead to less litigation? Our discussions with malpractice lawyers suggest the answer is no. In the words of defense lawyer Rich Mulligan, "In a lot of cases, it's more difficult to defend a doctor who orders every test in the book. That's because it's easy for the plaintiff's lawyer to ask, why did you order that test and not these other tests, and if you were concerned enough to order the test, why were you satisfied with results that were nondiagnostic." Which brings us to the differential diagnosis and knowing why a test was ordered in the first place!

Dr. Weinstock says that he has seen many "bounceback" cases where a test is obtained to the detriment of the physician. A patient who was complaining of neck pain got a CT of his spine that didn't reveal anything, so he was sent home. He came back the following day in cardiac arrest, after having passed out in the subway on his way to work. The autopsy revealed a fatally ruptured aorta. This is an extremely dangerous condition in which the aorta, the largest blood vessel in the body, tears open. The "classic" signs of this disease are chest and back pain, which he didn't have. However, the patient had unusually long limbs and a family history of Marfan syndrome—a disease of the connective tissue—which is a major risk factor for this disease.

"Some people took away from this case that we should have just done more tests the first day when he complained of neck pain and we would have found something wrong with his aorta," he says. "My takeaway is that we should have done a more careful evaluation that first time, and we would have picked up the warning signs from the history that there was something unusual about this guy's neck pain, something that was unlikely to show up with tests of his spine."

Dr. Weinstock goes a step further. "If you use the shotgun approach to tests, you're more likely to find something most of the time. But a lot of the time, what you find will have nothing to do with what's actually causing the patient's symptoms." And if it's legal risk that the doctor is worried about, searching down endless blind alleys can't be good. It's better to take the time to get the diagnosis right—and have a partnership with the patient along the way.

"Are you saying that there is no role for rules, or pathways, or algorithms in medicine? What about the 'checklists' that Dr. Atul Gawande and others have promoted to improve healthcare quality?"

There is certainly a role for protocols and procedures in medicine, as there is in most disciplines. Protocols can be very useful in the operating room, where meticulous attention must be paid to every detail—it's one arena where having standardized boxes to check off is a great addition to improve patient care.[8] The same goes for infection control: it's useful to have someone check off a list to ensure that invasive procedures are done with sterile technique.

The same thing goes for pathways. For certain diseases that require pro-tocolized treatment, like chemotherapy for cancer, or clot-dissolving agents for stroke, following a set pathway is a good way to reduce error. In his best-selling book, *Blink*, Malcolm Gladwell talks about how high-stress situations reduce the ability of individuals to make sound decisions.[9] High-stress situations are abundant in medicine, and there is a role for algorithms in these situations as a method to reduce error. A classic example is the use of "A, B, Cs": every paramedic, nurse, and doctor is taught in emergency situations to begin thinking of the Airway, then Breathing, then Circulation. A more advanced example is the use of airway algorithms. Dr. Ron Walls revolutionized emergency medicine with a variety of algorithms for managing patients who need to have an artificial airway placed in order to maintain breathing. "In these high risk situations, doctors are so stressed that they can't think creatively," he tells us. "Having an algorithm allows the provider to use a structured framework to guide their decisions and actions." We agree with the use of a proven, methodical approach in situations like stressful and high-risk situations such as these.

What about the role of recipes and rules in diagnosis? So far, we have issued a blanket *no* to a cookbook approach to diagnosis, but the real answer is a bit more nuanced. To get at the subtleties, we spoke with Professor Ian Stiell from the University of Ottawa in Canada. Professor Stiell is a pioneer in developing and testing "decision rules" around imaging tests—that is, rules to determine when to order X-rays and other tests.

"What prompted me to look into this field was that I saw how doctors ordered X-rays by habit," says Professor Stiell. "All the patients with knee sprains and ankle sprains, they didn't need X-rays to be able to say they didn't have a fracture. The X-rays were inefficient, so I came up with decision rules to help cut down on the number of tests done." These decision rules became the Ottawa Knee Rules and the Ottawa Ankle Rules, which are widely used in medicine today to help the physician decide which patients need X-rays and which ones don't.

We acknowledge Professor Stiell's reasoning and do think that these decision rules can streamline decision-making by doctors. We also support Dr. Ali Raja's and others' efforts to use decision rules to help reduce imaging tests—in part because all of these efforts are aimed at getting the physician to think about why they are ordering tests and perhaps to have more discussions with their patients.[10]

Another pioneer of decision rules is Dr. Jerome Hoffman, from the University of California, Los Angeles. He concurs with us that recipes in diagnosis should be used with much caution, and he calls such tools (including ones that he and his colleagues came up with) "decision instruments." That's because he says they should never be seen as "rules" that can't be broken.

"Some decision instruments can help when we're asking a straightforward, yes or no question, such as, should we—yes or no—do an X-ray of someone's ankle," he says. "There are only a very limited number of ways that a broken ankle can present—so if none of those are there, it's extremely improbable that we'll find a fracture . . . and therefore there's very little reason we should go looking for one. Most decisions are more complex than this, and then decision instruments tend not to work nearly well enough to improve on the clinical judgment of a *reasonable*—and I don't mean *expert*—practitioner. There are nine thousand ways a complex disease like pulmonary embolism or heart attack can present, so trying to capture that in a simple 'rule' is not going to be possible, and will likely result in a great deal of confusion."

What he recommends when faced with a "rule" is to learn from it. "If the decision instrument says, here are the five things to calculate, keep these things in mind. They're probably important and can help you with the diagnosis. But don't think you have to apply the rule mathematically or to follow it slavishly."

Our take on the role of recipes in diagnosis, and checklists and pathways and rules and algorithms, is to use them cautiously and thoughtfully, with a healthy dose of common sense. In the right situation, such as in infection control and in highly stressful emergency situations, checklists and pathways can be very useful, even essential. There may even be a role for rules and algorithms in diagnosis. For example, checklists can be helpful as a memory aid to make sure that all the necessary questions are asked, or as a final "gut check" after a diagnosis is reached to make sure that all parts of the history, physical, tests, and so forth fit. There is a big difference, though, between acknowledging the existence of recipes and relying on cookbook thinking. The pioneer of algorithms himself, Professor Stiell, would be the first to say that the presence of a recipe should not stop the thinking process.

To add a final touch of nuance: might there be such a thing as a recipe toward better diagnosis—in a sense, isn't that what the 8 Pillars represent?

"It seems like it would take a lot of brainpower to become good at this kind of medicine and actually provide patients diagnoses. What if the average physician just isn't smart enough to do it?"

Learning how to communicate with patients and how to make diagnoses is part of the training for every doctor. Every doctor has the tools to practice the personalized care that our patients deserve. We know this because the medical students we meet are perfectly capable of doing it, and actually it's only their later medical training that beats cookbook thinking and then cookbook practice into them. It's the medical system, which includes the medico-legal system, the financial pressures, and patient expectations, that reinforce cookbook medicine. Learning a different way is bucking the conventional trend, which takes mentorship and continued positive reinforcement, as it does take hard work, practice, and dedication to become expert at becoming good doctors.

For doctors already in practice, relearning a personalized, partnership approach to patient care will be difficult. It requires changing an entire mindset and approaching patient care in a whole different way. It is not a change that will occur overnight. The practice of medicine itself takes years to learn, and should be a process driven by continual improvement. But if the doctor is really committed to providing the best care possible to patients, then this is a change that is worth investing in.

We are confident that all doctors are capable of practicing better medicine. You, as their patient, can help guide them and give them permission to practice this better approach to medical care with you.

"What if patients don't buy into your ideas? What if they prefer to be passive consumers rather than active participants in the diagnostic process?"

We have more faith in our patients than that. Actually, our patients are the first to embrace individualized and partnership-based medicine. In our discussions with patients and patient advocacy groups, we have seen that patients intuitively "get" what we're talking about, and they are the most motivated to do something about it.

Pretty much everyone can recall being frustrated by the medical care system that provides an abundance of test results but no real answers. They don't want to go to a doctor who doesn't listen. They don't want to wait around for hours or days without being told anything, then going home with no diagnosis and no idea of why they had their symptoms. Almost everyone has a story about how they felt trapped in the ER, or the hospital, or the medical system itself. It used to be that patients have to resign themselves to this being the way it is. When they learn that modern medical care doesn't have to be this way, that there is a better method in which they actively participate not only in treatment options but also in the diagnosis, they are happy to be on board. When they see the impact on their care, patients embrace our approach to medicine.

It's not easy to go from being a passive participant who answers yes or no, and submits to tests to being an active storyteller and equal partner in the diagnostic process. But becoming your own best advocate is how you can make sure that your doctor doesn't misdiagnose you. Being actively involved is how you can ensure the best care for you.

It is our hope that this is how better diagnosis and better medical care will spread, from patient to patient, from patient to doctor, and from doctor to future doctors and future patients. This is our ideal world, but we are confident that we can make it reality, with your help.

911 REVIEW

- Our individualized, patient-centered approach to diagnosis saves time for both the patient and doctor. It results in thoughtful uses of technology, improved patient understanding, and decreased risk of medical malpractice.
- In this approach, there is a place for checklists, pathways, rules, and algorithms. It is cookbook mentality and cookbook practice that must be battled.

Conclusions

Thank you for reading our book, and for joining the growing number of physicians, nurses, public health officials, and—most important—patients who bemoan the practice of cookbook medicine and are incorporating an individualized, patient-centered approach to diagnosis into their medical care.

Finishing this book does not mean that the work is done. It takes practice to learn a new skill and to adopt a new mind-set. We encourage you to re-read the Action Tips and Pillars. Apply the Prescriptions. Practice the exercises in Appendix 2. Discuss this approach with your family, friends, and colleagues. Reach out in other settings where people need coaching on how to interact with their doctors, such as in parent groups, senior citizen centers, youth groups, community organizations, and patient advocacy groups. Discuss it with your doctor. Give your doctor permission to practice the partnership approach with you, and encourage her to practice it with other patients.

Thank you for joining us on the journey to challenge the conventional wisdom of medicine. It's time to take a bold step toward better medical care. You are the key to improving your own care and transforming healthcare for patients everywhere.

Appendix 1

Prescriptions for Healthcare Providers

Our patient-centered, individualized approach, with a primary emphasis on diagnosis, represents a departure from how many doctors and nurses are used to practicing medicine. From our discussions with them, most healthcare providers hearing about our approach for the first time are not opposed to the concepts, but are just not sure where to begin.

In this short appendix, we outline our Prescriptions to assist these practitioners in practicing the 8 Pillars to Better Diagnosis. These Prescriptions are the medical provider corollary to the Prescriptions for Patients we provided for patients in Chapter 14. Each Prescription is based on a question we have been asked, and we provide practical guidance for doctors, nurses, and health professional students.

We encourage our readers to give these Prescriptions and the highlighted ✚ 911 Action Tips a try. For those who are hesitant to change their practice, our recommendation is to incorporate one item at a time. Make note of your reaction and the patient's reaction. Try a different Pillar the next time. Work toward integrating the Pillars into a cohesive approach to medical care.

This chapter is aimed at healthcare providers, but patients may also find it instructive to review the pillars from the perspective of the doctor or nurse. As we have illustrated, understanding how your doctor approaches your medical care is key to your health.

Pillar #1: Tell your whole story

"I'm so used to starting every history with asking about the 'chief complaint.' How can I change this practice? Don't I have to start somewhere?"

It's true that you have to begin somewhere. But rather than beginning with a "complaint," why not ✚ *begin by getting to know something about your patient?* For just a minute, imagine what it's like to be that person. Who are they? How do they spend their day? ✚ *Allow them to tell their story* (without interruption), and keep an open mind about what is or is not significant, rather than restricting the conversation to one "complaint." Don't worry—when you put the story together at the end, the "chief complaint" will almost always be apparent (and the correct diagnosis more accessible).[1]

"I see what you mean about letting the patient speak. But I just can't! There is no time, and it's so much faster to ask yes-or-no questions."

It's a waste of time to ask inquiries that don't lead to useful answers. Yes-or-no questions and other close-ended questions, will lead you astray. ✚ *Probing statements and "how/why" questions actually save time,* and can potentially save your patient.

Here's an example: how many times have you asked a patient about how many pillows they sleep on at night or how many flights of stairs they climb? Have you thought about how this information is useful to you in any way, unless you have the proper context with it? So what if someone sleeps on two pillows at night, or doesn't climb any stairs at all—maybe she sleeps on two pillows because her back hurts and has bad knees and so doesn't do stairs. It's much better to ask an open-ended question that will actually provide information, instead of wasting your time with endless checklists that don't tell you anything at all.

"I don't know how to take a thorough history without asking very specific questions."

Of course you do. ✚ *Imagine you are speaking with a friend or colleague.* Find out something about the patient that helps you relate to their circumstances and their condition. Then allow the patient to direct the conversation, gently guiding them to expound on features of their story that seem important to the diagnosis. At the end, you can always follow up with a specific close-ended question if you feel that a critical detail of the history needs to be clarified, but you'll be surprised how infrequently you will actually need to do this.

"But there are really patients who are terrible historians. How can I get to know their story?"

It's certainly true that some patients have more trouble telling their story than others. The intoxicated woman or the older man with Alzheimer's may not be able to provide a "reliable" history in the conventional sense. However, even in cases like these, what the patient tells you (or doesn't tell you) can be important. Obviously, if the patient is unconscious, they're not going to be able to give you any history directly, but with these patients, there are other ways to get the story: from family members, from friends, from other providers like the paramedics, and so forth.

Most of the time, though, doctors refer to patients as "poor historians" because they seem to take too long to answer a question or they seem too unfocused. Very often, the history is there for the taking. ✚ *Instead of putting a label on them, hear your patients out.* Sometimes, a rambling history itself could be telling: perhaps the patient has undiagnosed dementia, delirium, or depression.

The ability to discern patterns in a patient's story and think in terms of differential diagnosis while conducting a conversation is a skill that takes years to master. But don't give up before even trying! Otherwise you'll never become the expert clinician you have every chance to be. ✚ *Spend more time with these patients, not less.* Allow the patient to actually tell their story. At first, it may take you more time to see patients. You may think that you are being less efficient. But in time, you will start to see the payoff. Not only will you become more efficient, but you will find your practice more fulfilling as you develop closer relationships with your patients—and you see yourself becoming a better doctor.

Pillar #2: Assert yourself in the the doctor's thought process

"This whole partnership concept sounds good in theory, but I'm way too busy to explain everything to patients in between the history and the physical."

Providing an explanation takes no more than 15 to 20 seconds. Surely you aren't too busy for that? ✚ *Use your explanation as a way to reassure your patient and to gather more history.* Rather than asking "Have you had night sweats?" explain to your patient why "night sweats" would be an important symptom to know about in someone who presents a longstanding cough and a history of weight loss. Rather than asking "Does the pain radiate to your back?" let your patient know that you're considering the diagnosis of aortic dissection. (You should also let them know that plenty of other less serious conditions can present this way.)

"Sometimes I really don't know what's going on after the history! That's why I'd rather wait until all the results are in before telling anything to the patient."

Give yourself more credit! Whether you're aware of it or not, ✚ *you must have some sort of differential diagnosis in mind.* From the moment you walk into a room to see a patient with "abdominal pain," you're probably thinking about some common conditions and perhaps some less common but serious conditions. Why keep it a secret? If you really have no idea what's going on before you order labs, you probably aren't going to know a whole lot more after labs come back either. The way around not knowing isn't hiding behind medical jargon and ignoring the patient. Rather, engage the patient. ✚ *Ask for your patient's help.* They are your best partners: chances are, they want to help figure out their diagnosis even more than you do.

Pillar #3: Participate in your physical exam

"I don't have time to do a full physical exam on every patient! That would take too long."

We don't suggest that a hair-to-toenails physical exam is appropriate for every patient. In fact, that would be as arbitrary as taking an encyclopedic review of symptoms or ordering a full body scan on every patient! What we advocate for is a focused exam, with the patient guiding the way to their body. ✚ *You need to explain to your patient what it is you're looking for.*

Especially if the diagnosis isn't clear-cut, this will allow you to pick up a lot of extra clues that might otherwise be missed. It will also be reassuring to your patient to know when findings are normal.

"How am I supposed to explain every physical exam finding to my patient? And what if they don't even want to know?"

We haven't encountered any patients who wouldn't want to know about the murmur you're hearing or the fact that you are concerned about their enlarged liver or spleen. We know you are busy, but ✚ *pointing out physical exam findings takes a matter of seconds,* and can greatly enhance your patient's understanding of their body and their disease process.

"A lot of people are squeamish about their bodies. How is it realistic to demonstrate physical exam findings on them?

It's easy: ✚ *ask your patient!* Say that it is your practice style to show the patient what you are finding on exam. Ask if that's OK. We rarely encounter one patient who doesn't want to know, and if you think your patient might be one of these, just ask.

Pillar #4: Make the differential diagnosis together

"I can't talk about the differential with my patient because I haven't thought clearly through it myself."

Well, that's a problem, isn't it? Buying time to think through the differential by ordering unnecessary tests is hardly the way to deal with it. You need to ✚ *learn how to talk about the differential with your patient* so that they becomes an integral part of the diagnostic and therapeutic process. Let your patients help you!

"As the nurse/medical student/physician assistant, I can't do this on my own. The doctor I work with rarely tells his patients anything about the differential diagnosis. Patients are confused and frustrated. How can I help?"

It's probably a good idea to first touch base with the doctor. Ask politely what he thinks is going on with the patient: can he explain the differential diagnosis to you? If you feel confident about it, you can offer your own differential and see what the doctor says. If he really has no differential, this is a problem. (Perhaps then you can offer him a copy of our book—or leave it anonymously on his doorstep!) If he has his own differential in mind but just hasn't shared it with the patient, ask if he would be OK with you telling the patient, or if he prefers to do it himself. Ultimately, ✚ *the patient deserves to know what is going on, and you can help bridge that communication gap.*

Pillar #5: Partner for the decision-making process

"The problem with this whole partnership thing is that these patients now ask me everything about everything. It's so bothersome."

They're probably asking you all these questions because you didn't explain it clearly in the first place. Your entire medical interaction should be a partnership. If you had explained along the way to begin with, they probably would have less to ask you at the very end.

"I tried to explain to my patients the whole idea of the partnership. They just look at me blankly and say, well, you're the doctor; you decide what's best. How am I supposed to respond to that?"

Just like you aren't used to the idea of a partnership, your patient isn't used to it, either! The blank stare you're getting is probably because it's the first time your patient is being asked for his opinion by a doctor.

When you get the look, you can ✚ *explain again your philosophy of medicine as a partnership.* Explain the differential diagnosis and the options available for pursuing each step of the differential. If patient says, "You're the doctor, how would I know?" ✚ *you can always answer back, "You're the patient, and often our patients know best!"* If the patient still insists that you make the decisions for him, you can do so—but you still have an obligation to explain the pros and cons and the risks and benefits, and give him the opportunity to express concerns and ask questions.

Pillar #6: Apply tests rationally

"How can I talk to patients about the differential diagnosis and using probabilities to decide the value of testing? This is a complex concept even for doctors, and my patients are not going to get it."

Give your patients the benefit of a doubt and try. It helps to have ✚ *set the stage earlier by establishing a partnership and explaining the differential diagnosis to them*. Then, use the concepts we outlined in Chapter 7, ✚ *talk about likelihoods*. If one thing on the differential is very likely, then the sum total of all the other things on the list is very unlikely, making any one of those things extremely unlikely. From there, you can explain how testing can help in narrowing down the list, and saying which things need to be considered and which don't.

If these methods don't work, and the patient still appears confused, ✚ *talk about how you would approach it if you were the patient,* or your sister, or wife, or daughter, were the patient. This helps to give additional context to someone who is ill and may not be thinking her clearest.

"I'm used to ordering the same labs for every patient with the same complaint. If I explain it to patients and offer them an option, they might say no."

As they should! Patients have a right to ask for care that is individualized to them and their particular story and presentation.

You should ✚ *try your best to tailor your approach to patients by always coming up with a differential diagnosis first*. It's unlikely that every patient with abdominal pain will have exactly the same list of differential diagnoses. Then go through and consider which tests are necessary for the differential you just generated. This will increase your chances of getting to the right diagnosis for the patient.

"I explained to my patient the rationale for ordering this test, and now they don't want to do it."

So? The problem is not *that* they don't want to do it, but *why* they wouldn't. So ask them. If the test were equivocal in the first place, perhaps they have a good rationale for it and you should accept their decision. If you really think your patient needs to have a test done you can try to talk them into the test. If they still say no, document their refusal. We don't force people who are Jehovah's Witnesses to accept blood transfusions; people shouldn't be forced to do tests against their will either.

"All patients want tests. My patients come to me demanding full-body CT scans. How can I convince them otherwise?"

We discussed in Chapter 17 how this is not true: in general, patients don't come to their doctors demanding certain tests. If they do, it's up to the doctor to make an accurate assessment of whether this test is needed, and what the patient had wanted the test for. If you determine that the patient, in fact, does not need the test, it's your job to educate the patient as to why.

✚ *Use the right language.* It sounds negative to say, "I am not going to get you a CT scan," because it sounds like you are withholding some amazing treatment. Rather, say: "CT scans carry a risk of radiation. Luckily, based on my evaluation today, you do not need a CT scan, for the following reasons."

✚ *Talk about the risk/benefit of certain tests and therapies.* If a test is really not indicated, you can emphasize that the best case for ordering a test is that the patient will know nothing more, while the worse case is, say, permanent kidney damage from the IV contrast, and cancer from the radiation.

Sometimes, ✚ *you may still have to offer your patient the option to have the test,* if they still feel that strongly about it. If the risk is not insurmountably high, and you have already tried everything to talk your patient out of it, perhaps the test will at least alleviate the patient's anxiety. We do not promote the role of doctors as gatekeepers to the nation's healthcare resources in order to ration healthcare, but rather, as educators to help our patients decide together what they have and how we can help them feel better.

"I'm the medical student/nurse/physician assistant. The patient just approached me and said she has no idea why she is getting this test. What can I do to help?"

As before, ✚ *it helps to talk to the doctor first,* because you don't want to increase the level of misunderstanding by saying something different from the doctor. Approach the doctor nicely and let him know that the patient is concerned and wants to speak to him when he has a chance—can he explain why she is getting the test? It also helps to ask the doctor to get clarification yourself; that way, you, the patient, and the doctor can all be on the same page.

Pillar #7: Use common sense to confirm the working diagnosis

"I agree with what you're saying, but patients don't ask me anything. I give them a diagnosis and they thank me, that's all."

We emphasize that medical care is a partnership between the healthcare provider and the patient. It is the doctor's duty to provide information and to involve the patient, just as it is the patient's duty to make sure they are involved in their own care. You can try your best to solicit questions from patients. ✚ *Make yourself available.* ✚ *Give patients time to think.* ✚ *Actively encourage patients to think through diagnoses with you.* ✚ *Discuss your philosophy about partnership and the importance of individualized diagnosis with your patients.* Providing an open environment will lead to a collaborative partnership, and you can do your part to creating that safe space.

"But diseases may manifest differently in different patients, so how come if one or two things don't fit, we need to keep on questioning the working diagnosis?"

A particular disease may indeed present in many different ways. That's why it's important to understand the natural history of the disease. We're not saying every patient needs to have typical manifestations of the disease, but you need to ✚ *be on the lookout for symptoms that don't fit with the disease.* Also ✚ *look for things that may seem like extraneous information that may actually fit in to the patient's story.* (That's why it's better to be thorough and start with a broad list of differential diagnosis and then narrow it down, rather than starting with one diagnosis and sticking to it.) ✚ *A "retrospective history" or even a final "gut check" checklist is helpful to make sure everything fits.*

At the end, it may take slightly more time to perform multiple reality checks, but wouldn't you rather come to the correct diagnosis than find out later that you missed something important?

"What should I tell the patient at discharge if I'm not 100 percent sure of the working diagnosis?"

Most of the time, you can't be 100 percent sure of the diagnosis. If you followed all the 8 Pillars, you will probably have come to a working diagnosis.

Let's say you are 99 percent sure of your diagnosis but not 100 percent sure. Perhaps you think it was food poisoning, but appendicitis is potentially a possibility, too, and along with some other unlikely diagnoses, that constitutes the remaining 1 percent of the probability. ✚ *Explain your degree of certainty (and uncertainty) to the patient.* Outline what you are thinking. Talk about the probabilities. ✚ *Give instructions that include warning signs of other possible diagnoses,* such as appendicitis. You have to judge what other diagnoses are likely from your differential diagnoses (yet another reason why cookbook medicine doesn't work, and why you should cast a wide net with your differential diagnosis to start with). Then ✚ *be thorough and clear in your explanation and instruction to the patients.* Patients will appreciate your openness and thoughtfulness.

Pillar #8: Integrate diagnosis into the healing process

"Doctors are not fortune-tellers. How can we possibly give an accurate prognosis to our patients?"

At first you may feel nervous about making predictions about the future; you may feel like you are putting yourself on the line. But no one is asking you to be a fortune-teller, only to provide your best estimates. ✚ *If you are uncertain, it's OK to tell the patient that, too.* However, in all likelihood, your knowledge of the natural history of whatever is ailing the patient is better than his. So, again, give yourself some credit. If you say: "I think in all likelihood that this is just viral gastroenteritis—a stomach bug. With twenty-four hours of rest and clear liquids, you should be feeling better. Of course, if the cramps don't get better, or if you start to develop pain in a particular part of your abdomen (say the right lower part) it may mean that this is something else, like appendicitis." Not only will your patient be reassured for the information, but on the off chance that he really does end up having appendicitis, you really *will* seem like a fortune teller.

"There are a lot of diseases out there, and I haven't seen the natural history of a lot of them well enough to advise on what could happen if a patient opts for different treatments or even no treatment. What should I tell my patients?"

The truth! Patients do not expect you to be omniscient. They understand that you can't possibly know every possible permutation of every possible illness. ✚ *Tell patients if there is something you don't know, and why.*

Is it because the natural history is so invisible that nobody can know. Tell them, then give them your best guess. Or is it because this is a disease that you rarely see, with treatment modalities that you may not know much about? Tell them, and ✚ *offer to look up information with them.* The advent of technology is such that this information should be readily accessible. Your patients will appreciate the extra effort you put into helping them understand their illness and their likely prognosis.

We hope these Prescriptions have been useful in illustrating how to incorporate a partnership approach to diagnosis into your practice. *As you become comfortable with them, ✚ encourage other healthcare providers around you to try the Prescriptions with you.* Share the concepts of this partnership approach with your medical practice. Discuss them at the staff meetings. Work with the other nurses and doctors, and encourage each other in the efforts. Emphasize the importance of partnership, diagnosis, and narrative into the culture of your workplace.

You may also consider to ✚ *let your patients know what you are doing.* Tell them why you are changing your practice to a more patient-centered, individualized approach. Show them this book; share the Pillars, Prescriptions, and Worksheets with them. Invite them to be your partners in coming to their diagnosis. Note the difference it makes in your relationship and their care. Our book is primarily for the patient and teaches the patient how to guide the doctor, but there is no reason why you can't adapt the methods and guide your patients instead!

---

911 REVIEW

- This book is written as a guide for patients, but healthcare providers can also use the Pillars and Prescriptions to improve their own approach to medical care.
- Share this book with your colleagues, and tell your patients what you are doing. Invite everyone to be your partners in diagnosis and in patient-centered care.

Appendix 2

21 Exercises Toward Better Diagnosis

Practice and preparation are the keys to mastering any new skill. Our approach to individualized medical care is a departure from how many doctors think; it's also a new way of thinking for the patient. In Chapter 14, we provided Prescriptions to address common scenarios encountered when applying the 8 Pillars to Better Diagnosis when you see your doctor. In this chapter, we provide 21 exercises for practicing the 8 Pillars now so that you will be prepared for your next ER visit, doctor's checkup, or hospital stay. Some of the exercises will seem very straightforward, while others may challenge you and take you out of your comfort zone.

We ask that you read through the exercises and choose one or two to start with. Every day, you can come back to tackle another couple of exercises. Take note of your reactions along the way: write them down in a journal and follow your own progress. The exercises can help build confidence and provide guidance for when you really need to have the right diagnosis.

Pillar #1: Tell your whole story

By now, you know well that the story, or narrative, forms the basis of our approach to diagnosis. All the other pieces of the puzzle depend on your being able to tell the doctor your story. Beware that this is often an uphill battle. The doctor, the nurse, the medical student, the tech—they may all steer you away from your story to focus on what they think is your "chief complaint." They may start to throw at you a whole slew of yes-or-no questions or close-ended questions. They may interrupt your attempts to tell a cohesive story. You need to practice to become better at telling your story, and also to become skilled at redirecting questions and deflecting interruptions so that you can make sure your whole narrative is heard.

Exercise 1: Think about the last time you were sick. Maybe it was the bad headache you got a couple of months ago, or the flu you had in the winter. Outline on paper the story of this illness. Give the chronology of events and include how symptoms started and how you felt over time. Put it in context; emphasize how the illness affected your life, by using simple language. Use our worksheets, both the basic and in-depth one, to help you. Now, try to describe the illness of a loved one: a child's, perhaps, or a parent's.

Exercise 2: Find a friend, a relative, or a coworker and tell them the story of the illness you described in Exercise 1. Share with them that this is an exercise for practicing being a better advocate for your own health, or just try to work it into normal conversation. Use the same mechanics as you did for outlining the story and make sure to include chronology, progression of symptoms, and the impact on your life. Practice using the worksheets in helping you tell your story. Note your reaction to this story-telling exercise. Was it easy to do? Did it feel natural? Did telling the story make you better? Did it clarify any points for you? What was the response of the listener? Did they follow the story line? Did they ask questions? Did they seem to understand and relate to what you were saying? How could you have improved their comprehension?

Exercise 3: If Exercise 2 was difficult for you, find another friend and repeat the exercise. Was this second time easier for you? If so, it may help to practice telling your story before your next doctor's visit. Does it help to use the worksheets? It helps many patients to write down the course of their illness and bring the notes with them to their doctor. Those who are visual may particularly benefit from drawing out, on the graphs, the progression of their symptoms. Still others may benefit from a "dry run" of practicing their story before seeing their doctor. Rehearsing your own story may seem contrived, but there is little time once you're at the doctor to get your story across. By the time you think of additional details, the doctor may have stopped listening or moved on in her mind. A little preparation may go a long away, and you should make note of what works for you and do it.

Exercise 4: Ask a trusted friend to play the role of a hurried and obnoxious "doctor" who keeps interrupting. Tell them about your last vacation: where you went, who you were with, what you did, how you felt, and so on. Instruct your friend ahead of time to be as rude as possible and to interrupt you frequently with yes/no or other close-ended questions. Practice deflecting the questions and redirecting your friend so that you return to the story. Write down how you felt after the exercise and what strategies you came up with to stay on point. Knowing which methods works for you will also help you when you are faced with health professionals who insist on pegging you with a chief complaint or bombarding you with dichotomous questions.

Pillar #2: Assert yourself in the doctor's thought process

We advocate for an equal partnership between the patient and the doctor. It is critical to establish the partnership early on, especially if the doctor is someone you are meeting for the first time. Even if the doctor is someone you have known for a long time, it is important to continue reminding him of your expectations of the partnership. Early on in your interactions, make it clear that you would like to share in the doctor's thought process. After you have related the history and answered all of his questions, ask what it is he is thinking. A lot of patients find this part of the process particularly difficult because the act of stopping the doctor after the history seems foreign. The flow may seem different to you, but stopping and establishing the partnership is critical to ensuring that you lead your doctor to the right diagnosis. The exercises below help to ease you into starting the conversation about the partnership.

Exercise 5: Select a day where you will encounter a number of friends and colleagues. Perhaps you can choose a social gathering with friends or a work event. During at least five conversations, work into the flow of the conversation to ask what their thought process was. This can occur as a colleague is telling you about a decision to accept a company's bid, or as a friend is discussing where she is going for dinner that night. Casually ask if they can explain their thought process for how they reached their decision. In the course of your social interactions, you probably ask something like this anyway to show interest. Practicing this type of questioning allows you to find the language that works best for you. Make note of the phrases that sound the most natural to you (for example, "so tell me, what made you decide to . . .").

Exercise 6: Do the same thing as above, but in conversations where the decision involves you in some way. Your daughter is asking to stay out later than usual; your group is weighing the pros/cons of hiring another staff member. Before they have a chance to ask you for your opinion (assuming they will eventually), state that you would like to share in their thought process. Ask what it is they are thinking and if they can guide you to how they came up with their decision. This is more involved than Exercise 5 because it pushes you to assert yourself in the joint decision-making process. Depending on your personality, this exercise may be easy or hard. Make note of your reaction, and continue to practice this until you feel comfortable asserting that you would like to be involved in the decision-making.

Exercise 7: Ask a friend, a family member, or a colleague to discuss a dilemma with you. You can either explain the exercise to them or wait until someone consults you with a problem. This time, you are on the other side of the problem—not as the "patient" but as the "doctor." Think through the problem with them. Help them work through the dilemma and come up with viable solutions. Your brother is trying to decide whether to go back to school—what are some factors upon which he is basing his decision? What are the pros and cons? How should he go about making this decision? This probably comes natural to you because you do this anyway to help out your colleagues and friends, but take particular care to jot down your feelings about what it's like to be on the other side of a true partnership. You should feel no different whether you are the receiver or giver of the advice. This is the dynamic you should feel when you are next with your doctor; you should aim for a similar degree of collaborative problem-solving.

Pillar #3: Participate in your physical exam

Being an equal partner means knowing what the doctor is looking for, particularly when the findings are going to be discovered on your body. Participating in the physical exam is an excellent way to be establish rapport and partnership. In our experience, most doctors would be happy to explain physical exam findings and involve you in the exam. The problem is that while some patients are quite comfortable with their bodies, many others are not and in fact feel downright squeamish when it comes to an exam of their body.

We suggest some exercises to increase your comfort level with participating in your own physical exam. As with the previous exercises, these may either sound like a piece of cake or seem insurmountably difficult. If it is the former, congratulations: you are way ahead of the curve! If it is the latter, start slow. You can move on to the next Pillar and return to this one if you wish.

Exercise 8: In order to understand what it means when a doctor points out a normal or abnormal finding during a physical exam, you must first know your own body. Take a look at your body in the mirror and make note of your shape, curves, moles, and so on. Then be comfortable with how your body feels. Women who do monthly breast self-exams should already be comfortable with touching and examining their breasts. This is an extension of the self-exam. On a day when you're feeling relaxed, run your hands along your face, then neck, then chest, then abdomen, then down your arms and legs. Make note of how your body feels when you press lightly and when you press deeper. If this is a challenging exercise for you, give yourself the assignment to continue to look and feel your own body every day for a few minutes during a bath or shower.

Exercise 9: If you have a willing romantic partner, perform the same exercise on him or her. Become comfortable looking and touching another person. See from a doctor's eyes what it would be like to examine someone else. Part of being an equal partner is breaking down inhibitions. The doctor has extensive training and experience in being less inhibited (while maintaining appropriate boundaries) with the physical exam. You can do your part to try to see what it is like from their eyes.

Exercise 10: Learn the basics of where key organs are on your body. Everyone has a general idea of where the heart and lungs are. Study a diagram to see approximately where your thyroid is, what side of your belly is your liver and spleen, where the appendix and gallbladder are located, and so forth. Develop a general sense of what it feels like to have an organ examined and know what organ is being sought when a doctor presses on your body.

Exercise 11: Ask a trusted friend or partner to lay hands on you and press, say, your abdomen. Practice stopping the person and asking them, in a gentle and nonconfrontational manner, if they can explain what it is they are looking for. Practice asking if they can demonstrate physical exam findings as they are conducting the exam. A nonphysician friend may not know what to look for, but this is OK—the point is not for them to show you a finding, but for you to feel comfortable asking them to demonstrate findings on you. As with the previous examples, make note of the terminology that you use and remember what works best for you.

Pillar #4: Make the differential diagnosis together

You can't be diagnosed with an entity that hasn't been considered. As we have illustrated, many missed diagnoses occur when the differential wasn't thought through thoroughly. Just as you need to be involved in finding the clues leading up to the diagnoses, you need to take an active role in coming up with the list of possible diagnoses.

Recall that the differential diagnosis consists of four types of conditions: good stories for common conditions, good stories for uncommon conditions, not-so-good stories for common conditions, and not-so-good stories for uncommon conditions. You can envision this as a 2 × 2 table:

	Good story	Not-so-good story
Common conditions		
Uncommon conditions		

In speaking with our patients, we have found that people doubt their own abilities to come up with a differential diagnosis. They ask us how they can possibly be expected to come up with a list of possible diagnoses when they don't have a medical background. The answer is that all of our patients know more than they think! You don't need a complex understanding of anatomy and physiology to come up with a list of some diagnoses, and you certainly don't need to have studied tomes on every disease to ask the right questions that will help lead the doctor to the right diagnoses. Our exercises here work to focus your mind-set on coming up with differential diagnoses and on asking questions to ensure that nothing else is missed.

Exercise 12: Think about the following scenario: your three-year-old child is crying nonstop. Use as an example any of your children when they were three, or if you don't have children, think about some other child you know well (your sister's? your neighbor's?). Come up with a 2x2 table for why this child is crying. For example, a good story for a common condition for the child crying might be a tantrum after not getting what he wanted; a not-so-good story for an uncommon condition (depending on your child) might be being upset at a bad encounter by a stranger. The 2x2 table should look something like the following:

Differential diagnosis for scenario: crying three-year-old child refusing to eat dinner

	Good story	Not-so-good story
Common conditions	-Tantrum after not getting monster toy truck for birthday	-Doesn't like what's for dinner
Uncommon conditions	-Appendicitis	-Man in the ice cream truck stole his money

Try to come up with at least five conditions in each category. Your answers may overlap somewhat, as what constitutes a "good" story or a "common" condition lies on a spectrum and depends on the child in question. There are no right answers here. The goal is to train your mind to think of as many possibilities as possible, and to not neglect possible diagnoses—even if they seem more uncommon or don't represent a typical story.

Exercise 13: Continue filling in the 2x2 table for three household examples. You can come up with your own, or use the following: there's a puddle of water in the kitchen; an important file for your tax returns is missing; there's a funny smell coming from the basement. After you complete your lists, do one more check and make sure you ask yourself the question of what *else* could be on your list.

Exercise 14: Now think of the last time you were ill and went to the doctor. Write down your story according the guidelines in Pillar #1. Now, come up with a 2x2 table for this story. You may have trouble with the "uncommon conditions" column. Ask your friends and use the Internet. Don't worry about right or wrong answers. You are not taking a test here. Rather, challenge yourself to see how many diagnoses you can come up with. When your list is complete, think about how many of these differential diagnoses you actually discussed with your doctor. Is there anything that could have been missed as a result of not thinking about one of these possibilities? How would you approach your doctor about it now, if you were to see your doctor for this same issue today?

Pillar #5: Partner for the decision-making process

Once you and your doctor have a differential diagnosis, the next step is to come up with a plan for how to narrow the differential diagnosis and come to a working diagnosis. The doctor is used to driving this process, and will likely tell you rather than have a discussion with you about the next step. At best, the patient is allowed to ask questions, but there isn't a discussion about how to proceed, what the different options are, why follow a certain pathway, and so forth. At worst, the doctor might not even give you a chance to ask any questions before you find yourself in another room getting an X-ray or blood work done.

We advocate for a true partnership in the decision-making process. For patients and doctors alike, this may represent a radical departure from what

they are used to. Our exercises here are geared to help you see what this partnership should feel like, and how you can achieve it.

Exercise 15: The next time you are having a serious discussion with your
partner, child, or close friend, take note of how the discussion goes and
how you feel. The conversation may be about deciding what car you and
your spouse should buy, whether your child should go to private or public
school, or how much leeway to allow your teenage son. For the purpose of
the exercise, the content doesn't matter as much as the process. Listen as the
other person presents their view and their plan. Note how you are invited to
contribute your point of view and how your opinion is listened to and regarded. Unless you have a some other fraught relationship with this person,
your experience in this reflects how you normally make decisions and
should feel very comfortable to you. Jot down your thoughts on this process
and make note of how you feel during the discussion. This is the feeling of
partnership that you should get when you discuss your medical plan with
your doctor.

Exercise 16: Involve a friend or colleague in this exercise. Ask this person
to discuss a recent decision they made. It could be a situation at work, at
home, or with friends or family, as long as it is easily explainable and you
can relate to the dilemma. Have them describe the situation, and go through
their thought process. Your job is to jump in and ask questions as a way to
assert yourself into the decision-making process with them. Note your feeling of discomfort when you first start doing this. This will likely be how you
first feel when you jump in and ask questions when your doctor presents a
plan to you. Unlike this exercise, though, which is not about you, your
medical care is about you, and you have every right to be integrally involved
in it. Write down what strategies you develop and what words you use to ask
questions in a nonconfrontational but direct manner.

Exercise 17: Now ask this same friend or colleague to discuss a dilemma in
an area that you have less knowledge about. Perhaps it involves an esoteric
hobby (should they go to Costa Rica or Guatemala for their annual bird-
watching trip?), or they need to answer a specific question with their job

that's in a field different from yours (is the merging of fixed income groups a good idea?). Ask them to start by presenting the plan to you. Use the skills you noted in Exercise 16 to gently interrupt and ask questions in a way that clarifies facts for you and also helps to get your friend closer to their decision. This is a more difficult exercise than the previous one in that you are being thrust into a different field that you may not know much about. That's the point of this exercise. Medicine may feel like a totally different field than the one you're in, and it is, in terms of knowledge base. However, the process of approaching decision-making and developing a partnership is similar. Repeat this exercise until you feel comfortable asking questions on matters that you don't know as much about. Be confident that if you help devise a plan for ornithology and finance, you will do just fine when it comes to advocating for your own medical care.

Pillar #6: Apply tests rationally

Once you have gone through the decision-making process, it's time to decide what (if any) tests should be used to narrow the differential diagnosis. As we have emphasized, tests are not always benign. There are potential risks such as radiation exposure and the possibility of incidental findings that may lead to further and more invasive tests. Tests often reveal no useful information at all unless there is a specific question they seek to answer; they shouldn't be used to blindly seek answers.

But how can you know how to apply tests in a rational and common sense manner? As with the above recommendations, you may not have as much knowledge on your doctor about the science behind tests, but there are some key things that you can do to decide, in consultation with your doctor, what tests to do (or not).

Exercise 18: Educate yourself on the most common tests. These include blood and urine tests (complete blood count, chemistries, liver tests, cholesterol panel, urinalysis); EKGs; X-rays; ultrasounds; CT scans; MRIs; mammograms; colonoscopies; and stress tests. You can perform an Internet search and look to see what it is the tests are used for. Educate yourself on what the test is, how it's done, how long it takes, what it's intended to show, and what it does not show. Take note of any risks associated with the tests, in particular the risks associated with radiation and invasive procedures. Having a basic understanding of tests will allow you to ask questions about the appropriateness of a particular test as well as how to weigh one type of test over another.

Exercise 19: Make a list of questions you can ask regarding any test your doctor suggests. These may include questions such as: what will the test show? How will the result change our decision-making process and narrow down the list of possible diagnoses? What are the risks involved in the test? Is this test necessary—what happens if this test is not done? Then think about the last set of tests you had done in the ER or at the doctor's office. Go through this list of questions and try to answer it for this last set of tests. Try to see if you can figure out the rationale behind the tests last time. Make a note of how you would ask your doctor if you were to be presented with these tests again. What language sounds most natural to you? Jot this down and practice it.

Pillar #7: Use common sense to confirm the working diagnosis

Once the tests are done, you and your doctor should have another conversation about what the diagnosis is. This is the time to perform your own common sense check. This is the "retrospective history" that we talked about: now that you have arrived at a working diagnosis, is there anything else you need to fill in to make it stick? Have you put the pieces together the wrong way, or maybe there are extra pieces that belong to a different diagnosis? The exercises here help to guide you to do a final check and to continue asking questions.

Exercise 20: Think about the last time you went to the doctor. Say you were diagnosed with a stomach bug. Make a note of all of your symptoms. Were all of them explained by the diagnosis? Come up with a list of at least ten things that didn't seem to make sense. For example, does it make sense that the illness has been going for two days? Does it make sense that nobody else in your family had it? It's quite possible that the answer to your questions is yes, that it makes sense and is consistent with the diagnosis you were given (for example, in the case of a stomach bug, lasting for two days and not having a known contact who is ill could make sense). Still, asking these questions increases your understanding of the disease and may bring up additional diagnoses that shouldn't be missed. Now, reflect on your experience: in retrospect, are there questions you would have asked the doctor? How can you make sure that you would feel comfortable asking them these questions in the future?

Exercise 21: Many times, the correct diagnosis is made presumptively based on the best evidence available. There may be other diagnoses that are possible but less likely. To be sure that you understand what the other possibilities are, you need to be adept at anticipation. To that end, you need to practice "what if" questions. Think about a time that you or a friend or family member was ill recently. At the time you left the hospital, ER, or doctor's office, you were probably given some kind of instruction. Make a list of at least twenty "what if" questions. What if you go home and develop more pain—what would that indicate? What is the worst thing that this could be, if your diagnosis is wrong? How would you know if that diagnosis comes about? What if your symptoms don't improve in a day? Or a week? Practice coming up with a list of "what ifs" with a couple of different medical scenarios and write down your questions. This is a good list to keep and use the next time you are about to end your healthcare encounter—they provide a final safety check for both you and your doctor.

Pillar #8: Integrate diagnosis into the healing process

Good news: this final pillar requires no exercises. This is by far the easiest for patients to grasp. Everyone intuitively understands that to begin the healing process, you need to have a working diagnosis. If you went through the rest of the Pillars, you and your doctor should have come to one or two working diagnoses, and you should know what things could be causing your symptoms and where to go from here. This is the stage where the treatment, and the healing, can begin.

We hope that these exercises have been useful in helping you understand and apply the 8 Pillars to Better Diagnosis. Do not be discouraged if you find the exercises challenging; they are meant to be difficult so that you can be as prepared as possible when you need the skills the most—when you are ill, when your loved one needs medical attention, or when you should ever need to be hospitalized. Practice the Pillars you have the most difficulty with. Become comfortable using the Worksheet Toward Your Diagnosis. Reread the Prescriptions for Patients. Write down your thoughts and reflections in your journal. The next time you go to the doctor, begin practicing what you have learned. The first few times, you may not be able to apply everything all at once. Reflect and write about what you did right, and what you may be able to improve on in the future. Strive toward the goal of improving your own medical care, in partnership with your doctor.

911 REVIEW

- Practicing the exercises now is key to knowing how to use the 8 Pillars for Better Diagnosis when you need it the most.
- It's natural for some exercises to feel more difficult to you than others. Skip these initially, but be sure to come back to them.
- Learning a new way of approaching medical care is difficult and takes work on your part, but you can do it, with transformative effects on your healthcare.

Appendix 3

Worksheets Toward Your Diagnosis

Practice your new approach to medical care by using these worksheets. We have two versions here for your reference, a basic and a more advanced worksheet. Use these in conjunction with the 8 Pillars, the Prescriptions for Patients, and the 21 Exercises. Our Web site, www.whendoctorsdontlisten .com, contains the worksheets in easy-to-print form. The next time you need to go to the doctor, complete these before you go and refresh your memory with them as you are waiting to see your doctor.

WORKSHEET TOWARD YOUR DIAGNOSIS

Complete before you go to the doctor

Your Story

How and when did your symptoms start?

_____

_____

What do your symptoms feel like? Have they occurred before?

_____

_____

What were you doing at the time and how did you notice the symptoms?

_____

_____

How have your symptoms changed, and over what time period?

_____

_____

How have your symptoms affected your life?

_____

_____

What is prompting you to seek medical care now?

_____

_____

What has helped/worsened your symptoms?

_____

_____

Are there other symptoms that are new?

_____

_____

Medical history

Have there been recent changes in your medical history?
Any new diagnoses?

_____

_____

Any recent changes to your medications? Have you been taking your medications?

_____

_____

Other aspects

Any changes to smoking, alcohol, or drug use?

_____

_____

What is your living situation? Any changes?

_____

_____

Have there been other life stressors?

_____

_____

Your differential diagnosis

What are you most concerned about?

_____

_____

What else do you think this could be?

_____

_____

General tips

• Use your own words, as if you are speaking to a family member.

• Being your own advocate will save your life. Speak up!

• Interrupt if you do not feel like you are being heard.

8 Pillars to Better Diagnosis

#1. Tell your whole story

#2. Assert yourself in the doctor's thought process

#3. Participate in your physical exam

#4. Make the differential diagnosis together

#5. Partner for the decision-making process

#6. Apply tests rationally

#7. Use common sense to confirm the working diagnosis

#8. Integrate diagnosis into the healing process

THE ADVANCED DIAGNOSIS WORKSHEET

For a more complete history when you have more time

Your Story

How and when did your symptoms start?

_____

_____

What do your symptoms feel like? Have they occurred before?

_____

_____

What were you doing at the time and how did you notice the symptoms?

_____

_____

How have your symptoms changed, and over what time period?

_____

_____

How have your symptoms affected your life?

_____

_____

Have your symptoms caused you to miss work or school? Have you been able to be excused from work/school?

_____

_____

What is prompting you to seek medical care now?

_____

_____

What has helped/worsened your symptoms?

_____

_____

pain

time

Make a graph of your pain over the course of time. Your horizontal axis can be any time interval (hours, days, months). Think of pain on a scale of 1–10 if it would be helpful or just as "not so bad," "bad," and "very bad,". You can plot multiple symptoms. Examples are below.

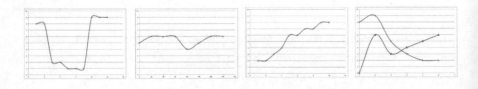

What have you tried to alleviate symptoms? Why did you choose this?

_____

_____

Are there other symptoms that are new?

_____

_____

THE ADVANCED DIAGNOSIS WORKSHEET

Medical history

Have there been recent changes in your medical history? Any new diagnoses?

_____

_____

Any recent changes to your medications? Have you been taking your medications?

_____

_____

Other aspects

Any changes to smoking, alcohol, or drug use?

_____

_____

What is your living situation? Any changes?

_____

_____

Have there been other life stressors?

_____

_____

Your differential diagnosis

What did you initially attribute your symptoms to? Why?

_____

_____

Is this still what you think is going on? Why or why not?

_____

_____

Did anyone urge you to seek medical care? What were they concerned about?

_____

_____

What are you most concerned about?

_____

_____

Is there something you are sure is NOT the cause of your symptoms?
What makes you so sure?

_____

_____

If you have had similar symptoms before, what was it attributed to?

_____

_____

What else do you think this could be?

_____

_____

Questions for your doctor

_____

_____

_____

_____

_____

General tips
- Use your own words, as if you are speaking to a family member.
- Being your own advocate will save your life. Speak up!
- Interrupt if you do not feel like you are being heard.

8 Pillars to Better Diagnosis
#1. Tell your whole story
#2. Assert yourself in the doctor's thought process
#3. Participate in your physical exam
#4. Make the differential diagnosis together
#5. Partner for the decision-making process
#6. Apply tests rationally
#7. Use common sense to confirm the working diagnosis
#8. Integrate diagnosis into the healing process

Appendix 4

911 Glossary of Key Terms

Algorithms: a formula for solving a problem. In this book, the term *algorithm* is used interchangeably with *recipe, formula,* and *pathway.*

Anatomy: the study of the structure of the human body and its component parts. In this book, we refer to what goes where in the body, externally and internally.

Attending*: a physician who has completed residency and practices medicine in a clinic or hospital, in the specialty learned during residency. Also referred to in this book as *attending physician* or *attending doctor,* the attending has ultimate supervisory responsibility over the patient's care.

Chief complaint: the reason why the patient decided to seek medical attention. The word is often presented in quotations because we find the term to be problematic: often the "chief complaint" that is written down is not in the words of the patient, and the term *complaint* itself could be perceived as being pejorative.

Cookbook medicine: a rote and fixed approach to practicing medicine, particularly when it comes to diagnosing patients. Initially intended to standardize medical practice and provide a consistent level of care, it often results in practice as treating all patients using a rigid formula. In this book, terms signifying cookbook medical practice include *algorithm, recipe, formula, pathway, and cookbook approach.*

Definitive diagnosis: the final, confirmed diagnosis. Contrasted with *differential diagnosis* and *working (provisional) diagnosis.*

Diagnosis: a disease entity that identifies the nature and cause of the patient's symptoms; implies a unifying or underlying explanation or cause.

Diagnostic algorithms: formulas used for diagnosis.

Diagnostic partnership: the partnership approach we advocate for that involves an equal role for the patient in uncovering their diagnosis.

Diagnostic testing: tests that are used to confirm a diagnosis. Unfortunately, diagnostic testing has been misconstrued as "ruling out" a problem, rather than making a diagnosis.

Differential diagnosis: a list of possible diseases that could possibly account for the patient's symptoms.

Fellow: a physician who is completing additional specialty training after residency.

History: the story of the patient's symptoms and illness.

Intern: a physician who has just finished medical school and is in her first year of *residency* training (called the internship). Interns practice medicine under the supervision of an *attending.*

Medical student: a student who has completed college and is enrolled in medical school.

Natural history of illness: the uninterrupted progression of a disease in an individual. In our book, this refers to how symptoms come together, how disease impacts the body, and how this progresses over time.

Nurse: trained healthcare professional who is a vital member of the patient care team. Depending on the practice setting, nurses may have a variety of responsibilities that include performing initial assessment, drawing blood, performing other tests, and communicating with the doctor and patient. In general, nurses do not practice independently, but rather under the attending's direction.

Pathways: in this book, used interchangeably with *formula*, *recipe*, and *algorithm*. Specifically refers to a list of things that must be done for a given chief complaint, for example, "chest pain pathway" involves electrocardiogram, chest X-ray, and certain laboratory tests.

Patient care tech: a member of the healthcare team who assists with basic duties such as obtaining vital signs, setting up for bedside tests, and assisting the nurse and doctor. May also be referred to as nurse's aide, clinical care associate, medical assistant, or clinician assistant.

Pattern recognition: the act of taking in raw data and drawing a conclusion based on the nature of the pattern. In this book, this concept refers to the basic framework for teaching medical students that involves recognizing a disease based on component, key symptoms.

Physical exam: the process by which the doctor examines the patient's body for signs of disease.

Physiology: the study of body functions, specifically what each organ does and how they relate to each other.

Practice: a process of learning that takes years to refine and perfect. Referred to in our book in the phrase *medical practice* or *the practice of medicine*.

Premedical student: a student who has not yet entered medical school but is intending to. Typically refers to undergraduate students, but may refer to any student with the goal of entering medical school (for example, student in a postbaccalaureate program).

Probabilities: the likelihood or odds of something occurring. In this book, probabilities refers to the likelihood of particular diseases.

Prognosis: the likely course and outcome of the disease. Prognosis is usually used to refer to the natural history of the disease for a specific individual.

Provisional diagnosis: another name for the *working diagnosis,* or the diagnosis upon which one initiates a plan of course.

Receptionist: a staff member in a clinic or hospital. Usually refers to someone with no medical background who greets patients and takes down their basic information.

Recipes: rote formulas for carrying out a medical care plan. Interchangeable with *algorithms, formulas,* and *pathways.*

Residency: specialized postgraduate training in medicine.

Resident: a physician who has completed medical school and is in residency. The term may further be divided into junior residents (year one and two; year-one residents are also called interns) and senior residents (year three and beyond). Residents are physicians, but are still considered in training and so still practice under the supervision of the attending.

Review of systems: a list of all the body systems and symptoms associated with them. This is part of the medical history.

Rule-out: a term often used in cookbook medicine that refers to the necessity of ensuring that a particular disease is considered and then definitively decided to not be the cause of particular symptoms. It focuses on what the patient does *not* have, rather than the real diagnosis. ("Let's make sure to rule-out chest heart attack.")

Rules: in our book, these can either refer for set formulas, or can refer to evidence-based medical guidelines.

Symptom: the "complaint" that the patient presented with to their doctor, for example, cough, shortness of breath, or chest pain.

Syndrome: a pattern of symptoms that appear together and are related in some way. For example, runny nose, fever, and muscle aches suggest a viral syndrome.

Treatment: the medical aid given to make the patient feel better. In almost all cases, treatment depends on having a diagnosis.

Triage nurse: in some ERs, this is the nurse who sees the patient first when they come in and decides on the level of emergency and acuity of their illness.

"Work up": a term often used in cookbook medicine that refers to figuring out why a patient has a particular "chief complaint". It does not say *how* this process will occur, and is often used as an umbrella term to justify a series of tests done without explaining the necessity of the individual test. ("We're going to do a work up of your abdominal pain.")

Working diagnosis: the diagnosis upon which one initiates a plan of care. Often the working diagnosis is the diagnosis assumed to be most likely, as a result, it is also used interchangeably with the term *provisional diagnosis.*

*Note that all job titles are as they exist in the United States. Other countries have different qualifications and the terminology may be used differently.

Notes

Introduction

1. Have you ever used an Internet diagnostic tool, such as WebMD? These tools utilize a checklist such that as you input your symptoms, the list of what you may have shortens. With the cookbook approach, all you find is what you *don't* have. Checking a box for "male" will tell you "you're not pregnant and you don't have an ovarian cyst." Whew, what a relief!

2. In this book, we use the terms *cookbook medicine* and *algorithmic medicine* interchangeably. These are the types of medicine that follow formulas, algorithms, recipes, and pathways (also interchangeable terms). Please see Appendix 4 for a full glossary of terms.

3. Learning the algorithmic approach can take time and effort to learn as well. In fact, some doctors devote their entire careers to doing so.

4. The World Bank. http://data.worldbank.org/ (accessed 23 August 2011).

5. 62 percent of those who filed for personal bankruptcy in 2007 stated that the cause of their bankruptcy was medical expenditure. Himmelstein D, Warren E, Thorne D et al. *Health Affairs*, 2005. Available http://content.healthaffairs.org/content/suppl/2005/01/28/hlthaff.w5.63.DC1 (accessed 23 August 2011).

6. The World Health Organization and the Commonwealth Fund release regular reports detailing the relative rank of the United States compared with other developed countries. The Commonwealth Fund 2010 report can be found here: http://www.commonwealthfund.org/Publications/Fund-Reports/2010/Jun/Mirror-Mirror-Update.aspx (accessed 23 August 2011).

7. Weinberger S. http://articles.philly.com/2011-06-09/news/29638875_1_ct-scan-testing-health-care-system (accessed 23 August 2011).

8. The Institute of Medicine. To Err is Human. 1999; available http://www.iom.edu/Re ports/1999/To-Err-is-Human-Building-A-Safer-Health-System.aspx (accessed 23 August 2011).
9. Ibid.

One: From Shamans to Black Boxes

1. Martin EA. "Transient global amnesia: a report of eleven cases, including five of amnesia at the seaside." *Irish J Med Sci.* 1970; 3:331–335.
2. Studies have shown that diagnosis can be made by history alone in 70 percent of the cases. Hampton JR et al. "Contribution of history-taking, physical examination, and laboratory evaluation to diagnosis and management of medical outpatients." *BMJ.* 1975; 2:486–489.
3. This appears to be a fairly universal concept across diverse cultures separated by time and geography: e.g., sangomas in Zulu cultures in Africa, Hatalli Navajo medicine men in Native-American culture, curanderos in Peruvian Amazon culture, Shi Yi in Hmong culture.
4. Don José Campos. *The Shaman & Ayahuasca: Journeys to Sacred Realms.* (San Francisco: Divine Arts, 2011).
5. Nicholas Tapp. *The Hmong of China: Context, Agency, and the Imaginary.* (Leiden, The Netherlands: Brill Academic Publishers, 2002).
6. Barnes PM et al. "Complementary and alternative medicine use among adults: United States, 2002." *Advance Data* 2004; 343:1–19.
7. Paul Ghalioungui, *Magic and Medical Science in Ancient Egypt* (London: Hodner and Stoughton, 1963), 58. Interestingly, Imhotep was quite a man of many talents: he is also credited as the creator of the papyrus and as an architect of many of Egypt's ancient pyramids
8. The Edwin Smith Papyrus labeled entities diseases, though to us today, what was called a disease is more like a presentation of a problem rather than a diagnosis—for example, they called head injury a disease.
9. F. J. Horstmanshoff, et al. *Magic and Rationality in Ancient Near Eastern and Graeco-Roman Medicine.* (Leiden, The Netherlands: Brill Publishers, 2004), 99.
10. In fact, Hippocrates's method actively ran counter to the other school of thought in Ancient Greece at the time, the Knidian school, that did emphasize diagnosis.
11. We will talk more about Sir William Osler in the next chapter on the evolution of training of young doctors. For more information, please see his book, the *Principles and Practice of Medicine* (1912) Available at mcgovern.library.tmc.edu (Accessed 26 May 2012).
12. Council on Graduate Medical Education. www.cogme.org (accessed 12 August 2011).
13. Even if they then get insurance, the worsening dearth of primary care doctors is such that the wait to establish care with one is often overwhelming. Massachusetts, where we practice, was the first state to institute mandatory health insurance, and the wait to find a new primary care doctor there is over a hundred days.

14. We use the terminology here with caution. Too often, organized medicine has attributed medical malpractice to be the major cause of all problems in modern healthcare. Fear of medical malpractice does indeed inspire some physicians to test more, but much of this fear is unfounded, and more testing is no guarantee against a lawsuit; in fact, more talking and less testing is the preferred approach, from a pure risk-management perspective.

15. Jena AB, Seabury S, Lakdwalla D et al. Malpractice risk according to physician specialty. *N Engl J Med,* 2011; 365:629–36.

16. Mistakenly, as it turns out, because jurors tend to show a surprising amount of common sense.

17. Some excellent Web sites on shared-decision making include: https://www.cahps .ahrq.gov/qiguide/content/interventions/SharedDecisionMaking.aspx and http://www .informedmedicaldecisions.org/ (accessed 23 August 2011).

Two: Do As I Say; Do As I Do

1. Markel H. "Abraham Flexner and His Remarkable Report on Medical Education: A Century Later." *JAMA,* 2010; 303(9): 888–90. 303.

2. Later in life, Flexner wrote on a number of other topics, too, including social work and prostitution.

3. The University of Louisville was one of the institutions that Abraham Flexner condemned in his report.

4. Medical training elsewhere in the world follows a similar trajectory, but there are significant differences in timing and content of training. For example, in the U.K., Russia, and China, medical school is an undergraduate degree that takes six years to complete. In these and most other countries, completion of a one-year internship postgraduation is sufficient to qualify as a general practitioner. Specialty training is not readily accessible to most of the developing world. Graduates often seek postgraduate training in developed countries, but the majority practice in a specialty without postgraduate residency training. The residency is referred to as the "registrarship" in the U.K. and in Commonwealth countries. A description of medical training can found in the following article: Wen LS et al. "Africa's first emergency medicine training program at the University of Cape Town/Stellenbosch University: history, progress, and lessons learned." *Acad Emerg Med,* 2011; 18(8):868–71.

5. There are a few combined bachelors-M.D. programs in the United States, such as the programs at Brown University, University of Missouri–Kansas City, and the University of Southern California.

6. Allopathic medical school is what one generally thinks of as "medical school"—it produces graduates who hold the M.D. degree. Osteopathic medical schools are similar to allopathic training, but also include additional training in osteopathy and the musculoskeletal system. These graduates hold the D.O. (Doctor of Osteopathy) degree, and are able to practice in generally the same specialties as those with the M.D. degree.

7. The piece of legislation that discusses this is known as the Emergency Medical Treatment and Active Labor Act. More information can be found here: http://www.emtala.com/ (accessed 23 August 2011).

8. In the past, a new graduate could practice medicine for a year and become licensed as a General Practitioner ("G.P."). This is still the standard of practice in many developing countries where postgraduate training is limited. In the United States, the field of medicine formerly practiced by G.P.s is now known as Family Medicine, and requires three years of postgraduate residency training.

9. There are some terrific novels on the experience of physicians-in-training. These include: Samuel Shem, *House of God* (New York: Dell, 1980); Perri Klass, *A Not Entirely Benign Procedure* (New York: Plume, 1984); Sandeep Jauhur, *Intern: A Doctor's Initiation* (New York: Farrar, Strauss and Giroux, 2007).

10. In recent years, resident- and patient-advocacy groups have raised the concern about the impact of these long work hours on resident well-being and patient safety. As a result, residency accreditation groups have imposed limits such as the 80-hour work week. This has brought up a number of controversial issues, such as how to balance rest and safe patient care with learning enough medicine during the training process to function independently after training.

11. Studies have borne out this contention, for example, in showing that those who ask a checklist of questions rather than asking for the narrative results in decreased understanding of the patient's symptom and lower rate of diagnosis. Dyche L, Swiderski D. "The effect of physician solicitation approaches on ability to identify patient concerns," *J Gen Int Med*. 2005; 20: 267–70.

12. Specialization is one more trend that encourages more narrowing of focus in approaching patients.

13. It should be noted that education does not stop at the end of the formal training process. Attending physicians are required to undergo Continuing Medical Education (CME), which they can fulfill through going to national meetings and taking specific CME courses. Doctors also have to keep up their board certification and pass nationalized exams. These are all further opportunities to improve doctors' knowledge—and potentially change their practice patterns. This chapter specifically addresses the training of medical doctors. Patient care is also provided by a variety of other healthcare professionals, including physicians' assistants, nurse practitioners, and registered nurses. It is outside the scope of this chapter to describe their training, but they are an integral part of healthcare delivery in the United States and elsewhere in the world, and we will discuss the care provided by nurses and the importance of it in later chapters.

14. Association of American Medical Colleges: www.aamc.org (accessed 23 August 2011).

15. Ludmerer KM, *A Time to Heal* (Oxford University Press, 1999).

16. Flexner A. *Report on Medical Information in the United States and Canada: A Report to the Carnegie Foundation for the Advancement of Teaching*. New York, NY: The Carnegie Foundation; 1910. Bulletin No. 4 Available: www.carnegiefoundation.org/publications/medical-education-united-states-and-canada-bulletin-number-four-flexner-report-0 (accessed 15 May 2012).

17. Ibid.
18. Ibid. His exact words regarding this third part can be found on page 59, when he referred to research and original investigation as "untrammeled by near reference to practical ends, will go on in every properly organized medical school; its critical method will dominate all teaching whatsoever."
19. Kenneth Ludmerer, *A Time to Heal.* (Oxford University Press, 1999).
20. This is an issue that also applies in nonacademic centers. Tarquinio GT, Dittus RS, Byrne DW, Kaiser A, Neilson EG. "Effects of performance-based compensation and faculty track on the clinical activity, research portfolio, and teaching mission of a large academic department of medicine," *Acad Med.* 2003; 78:690–701
21. For more on this topic, please read this article: Ludmerer K. "The internal challenges to medical education," *Trans Am Clin Climatol Assoc.* 2003; 114:241–253, or Kenneth Ludmerer's excellent book, *A Time to Heal.*
22. At HMS it's called "Introduction to Clinical Medicine," but it's the same idea.
23. Flexner A. "Scientific medicine in America—young, vigorous and positivistic—is today sadly deficient in cultural and philosophic background." In *Medical Education: A comparative study* (New York: Macmillan, 1925).
24. To address the shortage of physicians, new medical schools have been opening up, and existing medical schools have been expanding. However, the rate of U.S. medical graduates will not increase nearly enough to compensate for the acute shortage. The United States has been criticized for its brain-drain policies of recruiting physicians away from developing nations that have a much greater need for their healthcare workforce. Already, at present, one-third of all resident physicians in the United States are graduates of foreign medical schools. Proponents of this recruitment policy say that we are giving opportunities to physicians who may return to their home countries afterward. The statistics, though, tell us a different story: those physicians recruited away from their home countries tend to stay in the United States. For more information, please see the writings of Professor Fitzhugh Mullan, "Metrics of the brain drain," *N Engl J Med.* 2005; 353:1810–1818.
25. The George Washington University is conducting a study called "Beyond Flexner," which looks at alternate models of medical education, including those that are referenced here in the text. Dr. Wen was a member of the Beyond Flexner Commission.
26. Council on Graduate Medical Education, 18th Report. There are other factors, too, including mounting debt load. Dr. Wen was a member of the council and participated in the drafting of this report.
27. Wen LS et al. "Social accountability in health professional education." *Lancet*; 2010 (epub ahead of print).
28. Ibid.

Part II: Cookbook Medicine—Live from the ER

1. There may even be a role for recipes in straightforward diagnoses: testing urine to diagnose a urinary tract infection, for example, or obtaining a throat swab to check for strep throat. Arguably, though, these are not things you need to see a doctor for.

There are "minute clinics" in pharmacies staffed by non-physicians that serve precisely this purpose.

Three: The Car Mechanic with the Pulled Muscle

1. Depending on the setting, patients can encounter several other members of the health-care team. In addition to the medical students, residents, fellows and attendings, there may also be physician assistants and nurse practitioners. Physician assistants, or PAs, can practice medicine under the supervision of an attending physician. They function in a similar capacity as a resident physician. Nurse Practitioners, or NPs, are registered nurses who have completed advanced, graduate-level training in nursing. The scope of practice for NPs differs by specialty and location, but often, NPs are able to practice independently in the outpatient setting. For simplicity, our book does not reference PAs or NPs, but they play an integral role in our healthcare system.

2. We discuss in Chapter 8 the problems with the chief complaint, including the pejorative implications of the word "complaint" itself.

3. The whole concept of nursing triage was rooted in the history of emergency medicine. Emergency medicine is a relatively new medical specialty, starting in the U.S. only in the 1970s. Prior to this, ERs were seen as no-man's land. The only doctors who regularly saw patients in the ER were sleep-deprived interns from other specialties like internal medicine or surgery. Patients waited for hours and hours without anyone taking a look to see who was there and how sick they were. In many ERs, nurses took on the role of being the person to "triage," or to figure out which patients needed to be seen immediately versus which patients could wait. For those who needed to be seen immediately, it made sense to have a pathway that could be initiated without the doctor's presence. Thankfully, times have changed. ERs in the United States are now staffed 24/7 with doctors, and at most larger ERs, these doctors have specialty training in Emergency Medicine, a specialty requiring three to four years of residency training. Some ERs have a screening physician available to see the patient when they arrive to do the triage; some ERs are doing away with triage altogether. Activating a diagnostic pathway isn't necessary anymore.

4. There are four components to a malpractice claim: duty of care, damages, causation, and negligence. Duty of care is based on the presence of the doctor-patient relationship. Damages refers to the result of whatever negative outcome transpired, such as lost wages or pain and sufferings. Causation requires proof that the action of the doctor is what led to the damages, for example, the missed diagnosis of heart attack led to disability. Then there is negligence. This is defined as failure to meet the standard of care that would ordinarily be practiced by other doctors in that field under the same or similar circumstances.

5. Kohn D. *60 Minutes* in www.cbsnews.com/stories/2002/01/15/60II/main324476.shtml (accessed 23 August 2011).

6. www.imedicalapps.com/2011/02/ibm-watson-replace-physician-artificial-intelligence / (accessed 23 August 2011). This is not a new concept. Malcolm Gladwell, in his book, *Blink*, brilliantly discusses how human beings can have an instinct about things that is far more accurate than any combination of computer predictions.

7. www.pcworld.com/article/223329/doctors_test_watsons_ability_to_diagnose_ill nesses.html (accessed 21 January 2012).
8. Brown TB et al. "Assessment of risk tolerance for adverse events in emergency department chest pain patients: a pilot study," *J Emerg Med*, 2010; 39:247–252. Even if this study did find a correlation between particular demographic factors and risk tolerance, does this mean patients should be pegged into a category just because of gender, or age, or other factors? Let's say that women were more risk-adverse than men in general. Any particular woman patient may have a different risk tolerance level. This is our problem with using demographic risk factors and attributes to apply to the individual—isn't it better to just ask the patient directly?
9. Davis MA et al. "Admission decisions in emergency department chest pain patients at low risk for myocardial infarction: patient versus physician preferences," *Ann Emerg Med*, 1996; 28:606–611.

Four: The Mother of Two Who Had Trouble Breathing

1. The term *CAT* and *CT* are used interchangeably.
2. It's interesting to note that the incidence of pulmonary embolism is one in 1,000, yet this relatively rare disease is considered first over the likely and more common OSA.
3. Risk factors themselves do not mean that the patient has a disease. In fact, there is a difference between epidemiological risk (what is common for a population) versus incidence risk (what a given individual with a disease has). So most people who are smokers on birth control do not have pulmonary embolism, and most people with pulmonary embolism do not have these risk factors.
4. Brenner DJ and Hall EJ. "Computed tomography—an increasing source of radiation exposure," *N Engl J Med*. 2007; 357:2277–2284.
5. An interesting article about "hospital-acquired anemia" from blood draws in heart attack patients: Salisbury AC, Reid KJ, Alexander KP, et al. "Diagnostic blood loss from phlebotomy and hospital-acquired anemia during acute myocardial infarction," *Arch Intern Med*, 2011; DOI:10.1001/archinternmed.2011.361.
6. Dr. Jeffrey M. Kline has written extensively on the problem of the d-dimer as a test that is meant to reduce testing but that actually has the opposite effect.
7. Instead, the doctor assigned her a "chief complaint" of shortness of breath. Why, you may ask, was this assigned instead of her actual chief complaint of fatigue? We don't know the answer, but can hazard a guess: shortness of breath is a complaint he was familiar with dealing with, and has a ready formula—a recipe—attached to it.
8. Dyche L, Swiderski D. "The effect of physician solicitation approaches on ability to identify patient concerns," *J Gen Int Med*. 2005; 20:267–70.

Five: The College Student with a Bad Headache

1. The traditional standard of care is to get a CT scan of the head followed by a lumbar puncture if there is suspicion for subarachnoid hemorrhage. This is because up to 5 percent of bleeds in adults are missed on CT alone. Interestingly, the algorithm in

children does not involve the lumbar puncture—so if Danielle had been eighteen instead of twenty-five, she would have not had to be on the "pathway" for the spinal tap. One wonders how much difference there is between the physiology of an eighteen-year-old and a twenty-five-year-old.

2. Not that filling out an "against medical advice" form would have offered much protection in the court of law. If Danielle had actually gone on to have bleeding in her brain, one would be hard-pressed to make the argument that someone with that condition would have had the capacity to make a decision about refusing care!

3. There is a difference between pattern-recognition and anecdotal-based practice. Pattern recognition is the result of learning from a collection of experiences, whereas anecdotal-based practice draws from one case and bases clinical practice around it.

4. An interesting part of this Mortality & Morbidity conference was a discussion of how the ER doctors who saw the patient the first time actually considered ordering a CT of her head—at some level her presentation didn't make sense to them as a case of food poisoning. But, in part because there was no pathway to follow for "food poisoning," they ended up not performing the scan on that first visit. This case should be a reminder to consider each case individually, and to follow the clinician's instinct about the individual patient who is in front of them.

5. One might argue that if the attending believed she was capable of signing an "against medical advice" form, that he was pretty sure she did not have a bleed in her brain. After all, if someone really had bleeding in the brain, she would not likely be competent to make such a decision. That he was willing to let her go if she signed the form suggests that he really didn't believe she had the diagnosis after all.

Six: The Woman Who Fainted at the Sight of a Sandwich

1. For more on medical error, please see Chapman DM, et al. in Rosen's Emergency Medicine: Concepts and Clinical Practice, ed 6 2006, pp 125–133. (Burlington, MA: Elsevier, 2006)

2. Rhodes KV, Vieth T, He T et al. "Resuscitating the physician-patient relationship: emergency department communication in an academic medical center," *Ann Emerg Med.* 2004; 44:262–7.

Seven: A Crash Course on Diagnosis

1. Although, as we've discussed, there are sadly fewer and fewer master clinicians around for them to observe.

2. The traditional construct that follows the history and physical is the assessment and plan, in which the physician comes up with a summary of what is going on with the patient and a differential diagnosis, then outlines a diagnostic and treatment plan.

3. There are far more common causes of pancreatitis than scorpion bite, such as alcoholism and gallbladder disease!

4. For those who want to read more about esoteric diagnoses, we recommend Dr. Lisa Sanders's well-written book, *Every Patient Tells a Story: Medical Mysteries and the Art of Diagnosis* (New York: Random House, 2009).

5. This is also why doctoring exists at all. If diagnoses can be made so easily by a computer algorithm, what is the purpose of having doctors at all? Yet, by relying exclusively on algorithms, doctors have dumbed themselves down to the role of the automaton and made the entire profession of medicine superfluous. But perhaps we are speaking a bit too harshly here.

6. There are some excellent studies on misdiagnosis in medicine. The Institute of Medicine estimates that 100,000 medical errors are committed every year, of which more than a quarter—27,000—are due to misdiagnosis of common illnesses. Dr. Sanders's book and others discuss misdiagnosis in more detail.

7. We expand on this concept of how to be a better storyteller in Chapter 9.

8. Arriving at these probabilities is a matter of clinical experience and judgment. The majority of patients with benign, fast heart rhythms who then have the same symptoms occur have the exact same thing as before. In a patient with "red flags," such as a past history of heart attack, or old age, the probability would be adjusted accordingly. Similarly, if the patient appeared ill, the probability would also be different.

9. In addition to all of the issues mentioned, the false positive rate—the likelihood that a test will be positive even though there is nothing wrong—is high, even higher than the probability of the patient having the disease. This is yet another problem to be taken into consideration.

Eight: Begin at the Beginning

1. In an essay, topic sentences are generally written last, not first. If the focus of the essay changes, the topic sentence must be adjusted, too. This should be the same for the topic sentence of a medical encounter: the chief complaint.

2. This brings up a point we mentioned before: what patient would actually come in saying, "my chief complaint is diplopia and dysarthria"? The words were assigned to her by a nurse, and illustrates one of many issues with dependence on the chief complaint.

3. This case refers to what is called a TIA, or transient ischemic attack. Colloquially referred to as a ministroke, a TIA represents stroke symptoms that resolve in under an hour on their own. Studies have shown that those who have TIAs have higher likelihoods of progressing on to a full-blown stroke; therefore, it is important to identify if one has had a TIA.

4. The ABCD2 score is a so-called "evidence-based" prediction guideline for how many patients will go on to have adverse consequences after an event that could be an early stroke. Many clinicians use this prediction guideline; our argument with it is the same as for all such rules, that they cannot be used in isolation and cannot supplant the need for making a diagnosis.

5. Flip to the "diplopia/dysarthria" or "abdominal pain" chapter of a book and you will find in print, in all of its glory, pathways and lists of history/physical questions based on chief complaint. The more detailed textbooks may go an extra step and recommend some "outside the box" thinking: maybe diplopia could be from eye trauma or

right upper quadrant pain could be coming from the kidney or even from the lung. But this really just leads to more complicated, and even less useful, algorithms.

6. What happened with this patient was that the extreme discomfort of the patient having a distended bladder increased his vagal tone and resulted in a low heart rate. Other possibilities would have to be considered, but addressing the patient's actual concern would have taken his doctors to the right diagnosis.

Nine: What's the Story?

1. We are not saying that close-ended questions are *never* appropriate. There may be times when simple, factual questions, such as "What medications are you taking?" or "What medication allergies do you have?" make sense. As we will discuss in later chapters, there may even be a role for checklists to ensure that all the basic areas of questioning have been covered. What we are saying is that the patient's story itself can't be supplanted by a series of yes-or-no, close-ended questions, however exhaustive.

2. In a more sinister context, this has been called "giving them enough rope and letting them hang themselves with it."

3. This same analogy extends to the El Al screeners that we mentioned before, and to the hosts of *Car Talk*—all of these individuals realize that the best way to get the story is simply to listen, with a few directed comments or questions in between.

Ten: What Does the Story Mean?

1. More information can be found at http://stanford25.wordpress.com/ (accessed 18 March 2011).

Eleven: Help Me Help You

1. An important caveat is that the true "classic" story is not always as common as we may like to believe. Take appendicitis, a common disease. The "classic" story involves right lower quadrant pain and nausea. Assuming that they are independent, if 70 percent of patients have pain and 70 percent have nausea, the likelihood of the two together is 0.7 multiplied by 0.7, or 0.49. This means that less than 50 percent of patients with appendicitis will have the "classic" presentation. Still, classic presentations should be recognized and considered accordingly.

2. Tests may also be useful in excluding a particularly worrisome diagnosis. Ordering such a test to "rule out" a diagnosis should always be accompanied by some thought process as to what the diagnosis actually is. Otherwise, simply "ruling out" bad diagnoses quickly degenerates into cookbook medicine.

3. Hall EJ, Brenner DJ. "Cancer risks from diagnostic radiology." *Br J Radiol.* 2008; 81:362–378; Smith-Bindman R et al. "Radiation dose associated with common computed tomography examinations and the associated lifetime attributable risk of cancer," *Arch Intern Med.* 2009; 169:2078–2086.

4. Berrington de Gonzalez A et al. "Projected cancer risks from computed tomographic scans performed in the United States in 2007," *Arch Intern Med.* 2009; 169:2071–2077.

5. In short, CT scans should be used to either confirm or refute diagnoses on the list of differential diagnosis—assuming it even needs to be confirmed or refuted. A patient with sinusitis (inflammation of the sinuses) might not need a CT scan to confirm this, but a patient with a bleeding spleen does. A patient with abdominal pain concerning for appendicitis might need to have a CT scan to refute this—but not every person with chest pain needs to be considered for a tear in the aorta. These are the finer, more nuanced parts about making a diagnosis, and we mention them here as a reminder that tests should be done with care and for specific reasons.

6. Kristof N. "A Scare, a Scar, a Silver Lining," *New York Times*. www.nytimes.com /2010/06/06/opinion/06kristof.html (accessed 23 August 2011).

7. http://familydoctor.org/familydoctor/en/diseases-conditions/kidney-cysts.html (accessed 12 January 2012).

8. It is possible that one test may assist with narrowing down two things on the differential diagnosis list. For example, say we were most concerned about appendicitis, but diverticulitis, an inflammation of the colon, was also possible, just lower on the differential diagnosis. The CT scan might both refute appendicitis and support diverticulitis.

9. Hoffman JR, Mower WR, Wolfson AB et al. "Validity of a set of clinical criteria to rule out injury to the cervical spine in patients with blunt trauma," *N Engl J Med*, 2000; 13:343:94–9.

10. One could still argue whether she needs a CT at all. Might an ultrasound, which does not have a risk of radiation, be sufficient to make the diagnosis? Could the diagnosis of appendicitis be made on physical exam and she can be taken to the operating room to have her appendix removed without the CT scan? All of these are decisions that should be made with the patient as an equal partner in the process.

11. There are multiple references about this, including Siegel RM, Kiely M, Bien JP et al. "'Treatment of otitis media with observation and a safety-net antibiotic prescription," *Pediatrics*, 2003; 112: 527–31.

Twelve: It's Just Common Sense

1. Someone with a bad rash could have an allergic reaction as well as infection, so there may be two working diagnosis. That person can be treated for both of the working diagnoses. Other times, watchful waiting is enough, or he could be treated for one of the two working diagnoses.

2. This is not to say that in every case, a definitive diagnosis needs to be made. Take the example of the skin rash above. Arriving at a definitive diagnosis might involve a skin biopsy. But is the certainty of a result worth the cost and complications of an invasive procedure, when the alternative, empiric treatment (with anti-itch cream and antibiotics), is relatively benign and has a good chance of working? Or take a common cold. A viral culture could help confirm that it is indeed caused by a virus. But the culture may take weeks to grow, and in any case, would not change the management of the disease. This is the reason we emphasize working diagnosis and not necessarily definitive diagnosis. Many times, a definitive diagnosis will never be known, and this is OK.

3. The child in question turned out to have a highly dangerous condition of disseminated tuberculosis. This case is written in Wen LS, Noble JN. "Clinicopathological case conference: a case of a little girl with fever and seizure," *Acad Emerg Med;* 2011: 18(11)e86–92.

4. Because of this, puncture wounds are considered a "high-risk" in the medical malpractice arena.

5. The Internet is a helpful tool, but there is a wide range of informational sources out there and some of them are suspect. In general, we are proponents for as much information as possible—but please remember to use common sense in doing your own online research.

6. In fact, based on cases like that of Ms. Labo, our hospital has now instituted a screening protocol for all admitted patients that gets to the issue of alcohol use, in order to prevent alcohol withdrawal from going unrecognized and untreated.

7. It is unusual, though, for reasonable patients to show up in the ER for what should have been a chronic condition. Doctors and patients should ask, what about this was new or different? Something must have changed, or else why was the patient there?

8. In the examples of these patients with chronic symptoms who are finally given a working diagnosis, the working diagnosis is, by definition, still provisional. Both the doctor and patient still need to continue working toward a more definitive diagnosis. Providing a working diagnosis is not meant to provide complacency. In fact, it's the opposite. A working diagnosis simply gives patient and doctors a starting point and a direction forward to understanding and to effective treatment.

9. A good summary of these studies can be found in M. E. P. Seligman, *Helplessness: On Depression, Development, and Death* (San Francisco: Freeman, 1975).

10. Hahn SR. "Adherence to antidepressant medication: patient-centered shared decision making community to improve adherence," *CNS Spectr.* 2009; 12 Suppl 14:6–9. See also Wilson SR, Strub P, Buist AS et al. "Shared treatment decision making improves adherence and outcomes in poorly controlled asthma," *Am J Respir Crit Care Med.* 2010; 181:566–77.

11. After all, doctors are conditioned, from the time they are premedical students, to be "right," and it's hard for us to accept that we could be wrong—or worse, uncertain.

12. Dr. Lown and his foundation host the Conference on Avoiding Avoidable Care, aiming for solutions to the problem of avoidable care in all areas of medicine, and the transformation of the American healthcare culture from one focused on volume and quantity to one centered on value and quality.

13. We highly recommend the writings of Nobel Laureate and cardiologist Dr. Bernard Lown. His book, *The Lost Art of Healing* (New York: Ballantine, 1996), is a masterpiece, and should be required reading for every patient and physician.

Thirteen: The Eight Pillars to Better Diagnosis

1. Remember the Seinfeld episode where Elaine couldn't get help for her rash because she was labeled the "difficult patient"? There is truth to the comedy, insofar as this is a fear of many patients—discuss.

2. Lisa Tucker, CNN news. www.cnn.com/2010/HEALTH/09/30/bad.patient.save.life/index.html (accessed 23 August 2011).

Fourteen: Prescriptions for Patients

1. Timing (and acuity in particular) helps the doctor understand the urgency of the situation. The theory is that conditions that have been stable (e.g., headaches unchanged for the past year) tend to remain stable, whereas conditions that are getting worse (abdominal pain that just started this morning) often continue to get worse. This obviously has implications for the urgency with which diagnosis and treatment should proceed.

2. We do not have any personal or commercial interest in this Web site; we only mention this as one example of a personal medical information card that can be made and printed easily.

Sixteen: Diagnosis, Multiplied

1. There are many examples of new treatments that are later found out to be no better than the existing. Often, the new treatments may be detrimental. Drugs that are recalled, such as Vioxx, come to mind. For further information, please refer to Shannon Brownlee's excellent book, *Overtreated: Why Too Much Medicine Is Making Us Sicker and Poorer* (New York: Bloomsbury, 2007).

2. Weinberger S. http://articles.philly.com/2011-06-09/news/29638875_1_ct-scan-testing-health-care-system (accessed 23 August 2011).

3. An ultrasound is then the test of choice to confirm the testicular torsion, but the diagnosis should be made based on clinical suspicion—and the treatment initiated based on it (e.g., calling a surgeon).

4. For information on opaque healthcare costs and how physicians are not even informed of the cost of what they prescribe patients, please visit the organization Costs of Care, founded by our colleague at Brigham & Women's Hospital, Dr. Neel Shah. http://www.costofcare.org/ (accessed 20 July 2012).

5. Please see the *Dartmouth Health Atlas*, which is replete with data on how more invasive procedures do not lead to better healthcare outcomes.

6. Callahan D and Nuland S. "The Quagmire," *The New Republic*, June 9, 2011; 16–18.

Seventeen: Countering the Skeptics

1. The same thing would be done if the patient is requesting a certain treatment. Not infrequently, we have patients coming in asking for antibiotics for a cold or a specific medication they saw on TV. We don't just prescribe the medication because the patient asked for it; rather, we have a discussion on the risks and benefits, and indications for the medication. Thinking through diagnostic modalities should not be any different.

2. Our anecdotal evidence is supported by literature as well, as we previously cited with the example of antibiotics and patient satisfaction.

3. On the topic of satisfaction, pediatricians have been aware of these risks for many years and are extracautious about getting CT scans on their patients, and we are not

aware of parents being unhappy with the level of care their kids receive just because they get fewer CTs.

4. Commercial interests is a whole entire discussion, and the literature contends that patients are a lot more savvy than doctors tend to be about the influence of for-profit companies such as the pharmaceutical industry. Shannon Brownlee has written a fantastic book on the topic: *Overtreated: Why Too Much Medicine Is Making Us Sicker and Poorer* (New York: Bloomsbury, 2007). We also refer interested readers to the writings of Dr. Jerry Hoffman and Dr. Marcia Angell and to the organizations Healthy Skepticism at http://www.healthyskepticism.org/global/ and No Free Lunch at www.nofreelunch.org/ (accessed 23 August 2011).

5. Preliminary data from our institutions on this topic include that the doctors who order the least tests and spend the most time talking to patients have the lowest ER length-of-stay, meaning that foregoing testing actually saves both their and the patients' time. These same doctors tend to get the highest marks for patient satisfaction!

6. And even then, it is the context of a working diagnosis, for example: "we know you have a pneumonia, but we don't know what specific bacteria is causing it"; or "we found out you have kidney failure, but we are not sure yet what caused it."

7. Please see the excellent series of books by Dr. Weinstock and his colleagues. http://embouncebacks.com/ (accessed 16 June 2012).

8. Malcolm Gladwell. *Blink: The Power of Thinking Without Thinking* (New York: Little, Brown, and Co., 2005).

9. Ibid

10. Unfortunately, in practice, the application of these rules, even in ideal circumstances, only reduces testing by a small fraction. And under less than ideal circumstances, they may actually promote testing.

Appendix 1: Prescriptions for Healthcare Providers

1. We are also not advocating for the chief complaint to disappear completely! The chief complaint can be useful in communicating the headline of a patient's story to another clinician. All we're saying is that when you are speaking to the patient, avoid getting boxed in by having to name a "chief complaint."

Index